THE HIGH INTENSITY FITNESS REVOLUTION FOR MEN

THE HIGH INTENSITY FITNESS REVOLUTION FOR MEN

A Fast and Easy Workout with Amazing Results

PETE CERQUA

Foreword by Tony Escobar

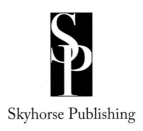

Skyhorse Publishing

Skyhorse Publishing books may be purchased in bulk at special discounts for sales promotion, corporate gifts, fund-raising, or educational purposes. Special editions can also be created to specifications. For details, contact the Special Sales Department, Skyhorse Publishing, 307 West 36th Street, 11th Floor, New York, NY 10018 or info@skyhorsepublishing.com.

Skyhorse® and Skyhorse Publishing® are registered trademarks of Skyhorse Publishing, Inc.®, a Delaware corporation.

Visit our website at www.skyhorsepublishing.com.

10 9 8 7 6 5 4 3 2

Library of Congress Cataloging-in-Publication Data

Cerqua, Pete.
 The high intensity fitness revolution for men / Pete Cerqua ; foreword by Tony Escobar.
   p. cm.
 ISBN 978-1-61608-844-6 (pbk. : alk. paper) 1. Exercise for men. 2. Physical fitness for men. I. Title.
 GV482.5.C47 2012
 613.7'0449 2 23
                        2012029211

ISBN: 978-1-61608-844-6

Printed in China

For my son Nicholas
Because everything we do is for our kids

Table of Contents

FOREWORD

As I look at the title of Mr. Cerqua's new book, I can't help but draw the conclusion that the title is catchy and that this book certainly does represent a revolution. There is no doubt in my mind that his message evolved from the inadequacies and challenges associated with the many fitness programs out there today.

There are literally hundreds of exercise and fitness programs available; most are based upon old, academic theories, which declare: "NO PAIN, NO GAIN."

Having had the opportunity to play two sports as a professional and to have also coached professionally, I have learned that nothing is further from the truth, especially when someone tells you that real fitness, flexibility, and muscle development has to be painful, inconvenient, time consuming, and costly.

I consider this book to be arguably the greatest fitness philosophy of the last fifty years.

I have spent thousands of painful hours in the gym and have had some good results. But knowing what I know now, if I would have incorporated Pete's philosophy into my fitness program years ago, I would have accomplished much more in a lot less time, and I would have done it without the burden of excessive physiological stress.

* * *

What direction is your diet and lifestyle taking you today?

Your body has 70,000 miles of blood vessels, about 80,000 miles of lymphatic vessels, and about 100 trillion cells. Our body is a complex engine, comprised of many mini engines within every cell! It is certainly unfortunate to see so much stress and so many people abusing their bodies with nutrient-poor diets and poor exercise techniques. It is also sad to see so many people completely oblivious to the concept of internal cleansing and doing exercises the right way.

Disease is rampant today, with over one million people succumbing to cardiovascular disease every year. In our country, there are over 1.2 million heart attacks and 700,000 strokes per year. This is not surprising, especially when you consider 237 million people in North America are overweight, 66 million are obese, and over 130 million people are afflicted with hypertension and high cholesterol.

Embrace this book as I have done; immerse yourself in it and incorporate Pete's exercise, nutrition philosophy, and his marvelous system into your daily lives. If you do this, you will get the results you have always been looking for.

Can you imagine losing those extra pounds of unwanted fat twice as fast? You posses that power with this book you hold in your hands.

It is the simplicity of Pete's system that incorporates and promotes, "result driven" fitness, super nutrition and internal cleansing, which makes it all possible. Can you imagine incredible health and an incredible body and doing it in half the time with NO PAIN?

This book teaches us about change, for in change we find the truth and the wonderful results we've all been searching for.

Mr. Cerqua is to be complimented for his initiative in having this important book published. Yes indeed, he has challenged the status quo by making available to the reader a painless alternative to the NO PAIN, NO GAIN philosophy ... and I absolutely agree with him.

Tony Escobar

Tony Escobar is a concept product designer and formulator of nutritional products. He has been recognized and quoted in many media publications in Asia, Australia, Canada, and the United States. He is a prominent speaker and is the recipient of special commendations and proclamations from the United States Congress, as well as the governors of fourteen states.

INTRODUCTION: THIS BOOK IS FOR REAL MEN

What is a Real Man?

A gentlemen, a boyfriend, a husband, a father. Someone to have a beer with on Friday and an occasional poker game with on Tuesday. A man's man and a guy's guy. The kind of guy that will selflessly help build that deck extension on your house or get the last minute tickets to Van Halen, in addition to helping you with your alibi. He helps with the 2:00 a.m. feedings and acts like a shuttle bus between sports. The best part is that all this is in addition to the first sixty hours a week catering to his first marriage, a.k.a. work. Hey guys, I know we've been dialed up to warp speed in recent years . . . the pace is staggering, and where we used to be second or third on the list, we now seem to be fifth or sixth. It's time to get back under control. It's time to take better care of the one tool that makes all this happen . . . your body! Hang in there a little longer. I am going to light the torch and lead the way. Let me show you some kick-ass options to getting in shape that will literally only take minutes a day. This program will recharge your batteries and not confuse you in the process. It's what you've been looking for to get rid of the gut and eliminate the back and shoulder pain, as well as pump up those "guns!"

Change Your Body in Less Time than You Ever Thought Possible

Why workout for an hour when fifteen minutes will do? It's not just about spending less time working out for the sake of spending less time, it's about getting a better result because you pushed your body harder. You can work out hard or you can work out for a long time, but you can't do both.

Stop right there . . . I know what you're thinking: *I'll just put the time in and work out for a long time because I don't want to work out hard,* right?

Unfortunately, it doesn't really work that way.

First of all, you will initially get positive results from your long workouts. That's because any new exercise program you put your body through will yield some type of result. But burning yourself out and regaining that lost fat is right around the corner, so don't fall prey to this common disaster we call "overtraining."

Secondly, your body will get used to the volume of work you are doing and resist progress. When it comes to working out, it is probably the thing that I hate the most. Imagine putting in more and more time each week, month, and year and getting nowhere. It happens all the time and I'm sure that you have gone through it yourself at some point. There are two things that we should all be concerned about when it comes to our health and fitness: building or maintaining muscle and burning fat. Reshaping your body is best done with high intensity exercise and weights. Reducing body fat is best done with diet—not with hours of cardio.

Are you a skeptic? Keep this thought in mind. Imagine you were a runner for your fitness program and ran five miles a day, seven days a week. You would burn an incredible amount of calories, but provide no muscle stimulation for any other muscles than your legs. Now, add the image of eating an entire pizza for dinner each night as part of your diet. Don't you think that at the end of a month on this program, even after running a total of 150 miles, that you will get fat? Of course you will! So if you have to watch what you eat anyway, why not do the type of exercise that will stimulate your weight loss, control your appetite better, and shape your arms and glutes the way you want?

Enter High Intensity Fitness

High Intensity Fitness is about getting the best possible result for your body in the shortest amount of time. Your home workouts—where you work on strength and toning—will fly by and your gym workouts—for putting on tons of muscle—will be over before you know it! High Intensity workouts are the solution for a long-term fitness plan. And when I say long-term, I mean LONG-TERM! My youngest client is ten years old and my oldest is ninety. Yes, you can build muscle and strength with this program at any age, even at ninety.

How Does it Work?

There are two mechanisms that are needed in any program for results: stimulation and recovery. After stimulating the body, everyone must recover so they can work out again and make progress. It's really that simple. One without the other never works and too much of either isn't good either.

Imagine these two situations: working out for an hour a day but not very hard and working out for twenty minutes a day, but very intensely. Neither situation is good. The first type of workout is low intensity, high volume. The workouts themselves are not very stimulating to the body so your body won't change. The second workout is high intensity, but done too often so that there is not enough recovery for continued progress. The best scenario involves balancing the intensity of the workout with proper recovery time to avoid burnout and make consistent progress.

With High Intensity Fitness, we will balance the intensity of the workouts with your recovery time. Your body will never get accustomed to the workouts and overtraining or burning yourself out is not an option.

Increasing the intensity of a workout can come in different forms. Slowing down the speed in which you lift weights will create more tension on the muscle, thereby increasing the intensity of the workout. Working a set to the point where you can't do another rep is more intense than just doing a predetermined number of reps. Running 100 yards as fast as you can is more intense than running a slow mile. In the pages ahead, I put together some High Intensity workouts that are very effective, but most importantly, completely doable for any man.

From home workouts to gym workouts.

From cardio workouts to abdominal workouts. It's all here.

There will be workout techniques that you may not have heard of to increase your intensity, like holding a weight motionless (static exercise) or lowering a weight but not lifting it (negative only exercise). How to arrange these techniques within the workout, get the most from your cardio workouts, and coordinate your schedule will also be laid out for you.

CHAPTER ONE:
TOP 10 REASONS WHY SHORT
WORKOUTS ARE BETTER

10. Less Time

Who has time these days? I know I don't.

Let me explain it to you the same way I explain it to my clients when they come in for a workout with me. What if I was your money manager and you gave me your life savings to invest for you? A year goes by and I give you my annual report and you have exactly the same amount of money as you did last year (minus my commission, of course). What would you do? I imagine you would fire me and throw me out of your house! This is what your low intensity, high volume workout is doing for you—nothing, zilch, nada. Be honest, did you lose a lot of weight in the past year with your workout program?

Any at all?

Did your strength increase?

If the answer is no, then you have to increase your intensity and be more scientific about your workouts and diet. High Intensity Fitness will yield results each week in a fraction of the time. The net result will be a better fitness portfolio in less time.

9. Actual Results

With High Intensity Fitness, you can see tangible results each week. It's very important to know that increases in strength and endurance always precede a change in the body. So you'll notice that the numbers on your workout chart will go up for a few weeks before you see a physical change in the mirror. <u>Please be patient . . . it will happen.</u> Research shows that an increase in strength and muscle helps the body burn more fat throughout the day at a higher success rate than hours on the treadmill, elliptical, or spin class . . . and we all want to spend less time getting what we want.

8. Very Interesting

How difficult is it to get on the treadmill or elliptical for an hour each day knowing that the only thing you get when you're finished is more laundry to do? It must be exhausting. That's why there is a new fad each year to keep you interested. How are we going to make these people come in and sweat for an hour and charge them money and NOT improve their strength and health? This is what the big gyms are banging their heads about each year . . . how to suck you in. First it was step class, then it was kickboxing, then it was some sort of boot camp.... My favorite is when they dig up something from 200 years ago that didn't work and try to sell it to you again (see kettlebells). Don't get me wrong. I am not against activities outside of your High Intensity workouts. I tell my clients to go for a hike, climb a rock wall, or do your Lance Armstrong impersonation if you need to get out and release some tension. But don't confuse these activities with result-producing exercise. High Intensity Fitness is based on scientific principles that will stimulate your body as well as your mind.

7. Based On Science

Haven't you ever asked yourself "why?" As in,

"Why do we need to walk on the treadmill for an hour?"

"Why not 46 minutes?"

"Why do we have to do three sets of 12-15 on everything?"

"Why not four sets or 37 reps per set?"

Well, I asked these questions years ago and wanted answers. Fortunately for me, there was someone who was blazing the High Intensity Fitness trail when I was looking for help. His name was Arthur Jones, who is the inventor of Nautilus. Arthur was an in-your-face kind of guy that wanted answers to all the strength training and exercise question . . . and got them. **You only need to do one set of an exercise if performed properly-not three or five. Only the simple-minded spent hours in the gym when 20 minutes would do.** Yes, Arthur paved the way. So instead of mindlessly going to the gym and doing "whatever," we now know that results come from a carefully planned High Intensity session . . . and it didn't stop there. More articles and research are surfacing each month. A recent article from the *New York Times* informed readers about research performed at McMaster University in Hamilton, Ontario, that showed a 30-second High Intensity workout was more productive than a 30-minute moderate intensity workout! I have read many articles like this over the last few years as more and more information has come to light. Hey, there was a time when we had to rub two sticks together to make fire. Now you just "flick your Bic," and voilà!

We have come a long way in the fitness industry. The "do as much as possible in hopes that something will work" method is outdated. The more specific and scientific methods are in. In my first book, *The 90-Second Fitness Solution*, I cited many studies to prove the effectiveness of High Intensity workouts. With this book however, I promise not to bore you with too much explanation of why it works, and instead just get you right to the workouts as quickly as possible.

6. Get in the Best Shape of Your Life

Hey guys, we make more testosterone than girls do. Yes, they make as much money, endure more pain, and are definitely the more attractive of the species, but WE make more testosterone . . . so there! Why should you care? Because it's the high levels of testosterone in your body that make for bigger muscles. That's why some people (both men and women) take steroids. High Intensity Fitness has a different effect on our bodies than that of our feminine counterparts. When the girls do High Intensity workouts, they get smaller, tighter, and stronger. When we do them, we gain mass. Wait, it gets better. High Intensity workouts promote an increase in testosterone, which is just the opposite of long, low intensity workouts. Hit it hard, be brief, and get the body you've always wanted!

5. Get Strong, Get Ripped

The stronger you get, the leaner you get. Think of your body as an engine. A weak engine will not be able to gobble up and use much gas. With a car, the excess gas just sits in the tank; but with humans, the excess gas (or calories) are stored as fat. Really ugly, never where you want it, always trying to hide it, FAT! A stronger body burns more calories than a weaker one. High Intensity workouts strengthen and tone the body where low intensity, high volume workouts do not.

4. Increased Metabolism

Check this out: Muscle burns 25 percent more calories than fat. So guess which one you want more of? That means you can burn more calories by lying on a beach chair while your buddy is doing hours of cardio. Burning calories while doing nothing beats exercising any day of the week!

3. Stronger Bones

Research shows that strength training can increase bone density up to 13 percent in only six months. High Intensity Strength Training does an even better job. My recommendation for avoiding osteoporosis and standing up straight all your life is to hit the weights the High Intensity way. Yes, even men suffer from osteoporosis. (While 44 million Americans suffer from osteoporosis, more than 14 million of those are men.[1])

2. Prevent Arthritis

There is nothing wrong with building muscle and changing the shape of your body, but your High Intensity Fitness workouts will also strengthen your connective tissues, which will in turn increase future joint stability. Having stable joints not only helps prevent injuries, but also helps those

---

[1]   www.osteometer.com

that suffer from arthritis. It's all about quality of life. With your stronger body, everyday activities become easier, and makes life more enjoyable.

And the number one reason that short workouts are better than long ones…

1. The Gun Show

Look guys, workout on the treadmill and elliptical all you want. Lift your baby weights and endure all the gimmicky stuff you see on TV, but only a High Intensity workout will give you the guns worthy of a "Gun Show." The kind of guns that will make the girls look and the guys jealous . . . and the workouts take less than 15 minutes!

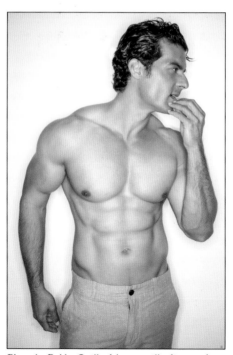

Photo by Bobby Quillard (www.quillardinc.com)

Stefan Pinto is a professional model and author of *Fat-to-Fit: 50 Easy Ways to Lose Weight* (facebook.com/stefan.pinto).

CHAPTER TWO: GETTING STARTED

Believe it or not, a great way to start your exercise program is with a garbage bag and your wallet. Let's face it, your old habits are not working for you (and if they were, you wouldn't be reading this book). So we have to start with a clean slate. That means getting rid of everything that is holding you back.

Clean Out Your Refrigerator

Walk into the kitchen and open up your refrigerator and cupboards. What do you see? It's all the things that were making you fat. It's time to get rid of it and make room for the good stuff. I know that in some cases you may think you are eating healthy, but in reality, you probably aren't.

If it's processed, made of white flour, or white sugar, **toss it.**

If it has a high amount of sodium, **pitch it.**

If it has gluten, give it the **boot!**

Let me guess, the only thing left is the baking soda and a few ice cubes. Time to restock.

Go Shopping for Real Food

Eating healthy and losing body fat is not about the latest fad diet or the processed and packaged garbage that's on TV. It's about real food.

- Fresh fruits and vegetables.
- Free range chicken and eggs that are high in omega-3 fatty acids.
- If you eat beef, get it from grass-fed cows only.
- Fish? Wild Alaskan salmon is best.

Now look at your refrigerator and cupboards. We haven't counted a calorie or restricted a food group, but you can already see that this is going to work. It feels right, doesn't it? By the way, chocolate is food and beer is not. There will definitely be room in your eating plan for a slip up once in a while, but we will keep it to a minimum.

High Intensity Tip

Listen, people slip up, it happens. The most important thing is rather than letting it be an excuse to quit eating healthy, take it in stride and continue your healthy ways. There's no reason to throw away all your hard work if you have a chocolate bar or two. Acknowledge that it wasn't your best eating day and that you'll vow to do better tomorrow.

Order Your Supplements Online

No diet gives us everything we need. Even some of my raw vegan friends supplement their diets. Maybe your joints are giving you a hard time and you need some MSM? A good protein supplement will make at least one of your meals more convenient. Most people I know need B vitamins for stress and metabolism. How about a cleanse? It's probably about time for you to clean out your system and give it the clean slate that you just gave your kitchen. I recently started using Isagenix products myself and love the convenience and results. It's the one–stop shopping that always gets my attention, but the key is that their protein powder comes from grass-fed cows in New Zealand. Believe me, cows that enjoy clean living are better for us then when they are lined up by the thousands and fed garbage that I wouldn't give to a rat. I will point you in the right direction and get you set up with anything you need in the High Intensity Nutrition chapter.

Be Prepared to Work Outside of Your Comfort Zone

This is mental prep. You will have to work harder and smarter to abandon what I call the "low intensity attitude." What I mean here is you probably think that since you don't want to work hard, you can bypass the lack of effort with working out longer. That couldn't be further from the truth. If it worked that way, we wouldn't have an obesity epidemic in our country.

So I'm telling you right now that you will have to put some effort into these brief and infrequent workouts to get something out of them. I understand that this will most likely be a little out of you comfort zone, but that's okay. You will embrace it after a while and will not know how you endured those mindless, lengthy sessions that you tried in the past.

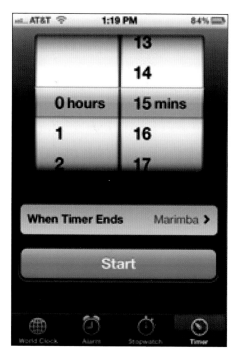

It only takes minutes to get started!

CHAPTER THREE: GET YOUR BASELINE

So workout-wise, how do we get started? How can I possibly give you a workout routine without knowing what your current situation and strength level is?

Easy. If you just spend the first week gathering vital information about yourself, we will have the tools to make these workouts effective right from the first session. The best part is that the information gathering stage is a workout in itself, so you will get something out of it as well.

Home Workout Challenge

As you start your exercise routine, you may not be interested in venturing out to the gym just yet, so I have some home workout options for you that involve little or no equipment. But first, let's see what your strength level is.

The 90-Second Fitness Challenge

This was a featured workout in my first book, *The 90-Second Fitness Solution*, and you can also find it on my website: petecerqua.com. The challenge is made up of two exercises: the wall sit and the plank. They are really easy to try. Refer to the photos below to make sure you have the proper form. Your goal is to hold each position for up to 90 seconds. It sounds easy, but wait till you try it. Even advanced people email me to say how they found it to be more challenging than they initially thought. The two exercises in the challenge utilize a static contraction protocol or "no movement." I use this technique as a great way to introduce High Intensity workouts to people who have never tried it before. In this situation, the static contraction will benefit you in two different ways. The first is concerning the wall sit. The wall sit is the static version of a squat. Try this:

- Stand with your feet shoulder width apart.
- Put your arms straight out in front of you for balance and do a deep knee bend or squat.

- Go down to the 90 degree position or until your thighs are parallel to the floor.
- Do 12 reps and let's assess how you feel.

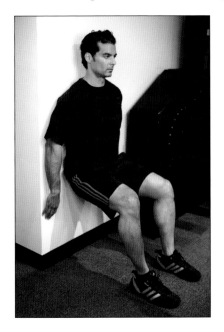

Basic Wall Sit: Try to hold this position for 90 seconds.

Did it get your heart rate up? Sure, a little, but the most demanding or important part of that exercise was the bottom part . . . and you didn't spend very much time there. Since it's a bodyweight exercise with no additional resistance, there is very little value or benefit in strengthening and reshaping your thighs. The solution for this is to get against a wall and do a wall sit.

What do you feel? Your thighs are burning, aren't they? You are getting right to the best part of the exercise and targeting your thighs with no movement. The other great thing about statics is apparent when we do the **plank**.

How many of you can do 10 perfect pushups or more? Those who are able to do a lot of pushups will benefit from the more advanced routines in the other chapters, but those of you that can't do that many or want to spice up your routine will benefit greatly from the static plank in the meantime. Either way, I am challenging you to try it out and see how you stack up.

So, how long did you hold each exercise for?

Over the years, I have found that if you can hold each exercise for:

- 30 seconds or less, your strength is below average and needs work;
- 30 to 60 seconds, your strength is average but you could use more;

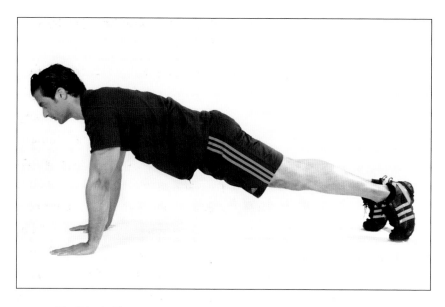

The Plank: Try to hold this position for 90 seconds after the wall sit.

- 60 to 90 seconds, your strength is above average—good job!
- Just made it to 90 seconds? You are "entry level" strong;
- 90 seconds easily, you are in great shape and ready for the next level.

If your strength needs work, consider trying the home workouts until you master them. As soon as you do, get your "gym numbers" and move on to higher intensity workouts.

Get Your Gym Numbers

If you are not interested in the home workout, in better shape than the home workout, or just can't wait to do the High Intensity gym workouts, then it's time to get your gym numbers. What are your gym numbers? Simply put, we need to know where your strength level is at on some basic exercises and apply that information to your workouts.

Our goal is to find your 12 rep max on the exercises we choose and work from there.

12 Reps Will Get the Job Done

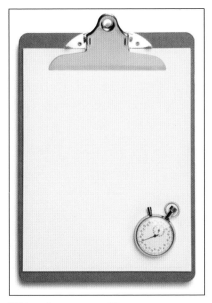

Write down your 12 rep max sets—make sure to keep accurate records.

I have chosen the 12 rep max for a few reasons. The first is that studies show us that it is not necessarily the number of reps that stimulate the muscle, but the amount of time spent working during the set. The optimal amount of time spent on a single High Intensity set should be somewhere between 40 and 70 seconds. I have always believed that if you can spend 90 seconds on a set, then you have stimulated the muscle sufficiently and are ready for the next level. Now, at my gym in New York City, I would coach you through each set until you reached the appropriate amount of time. But seeing as I'm not there with you right now, I'll have to show you a simpler way to get this done by yourself. All you need to do is a 12 rep set that challenges you for the last few reps and your time will fall right in line with the time we need to get a response from your muscles.

Let's take a chest press machine for example. You set the machine up for your height and do a light set of 12 reps. Since the weight is light, you should be able to do 12 continuous reps in good form with no hesitation. Because the weight is light and not challenging, it will not be classified as a High Intensity set and will only take about 12-15 seconds to complete. No problem so far, right?

For the next set, you will add some weight and start again after a minute or two of rest. What we are looking for is a set that goes like this:

- You push out the first rep slowly and very controlled.
- The next four or five reps are moving smoothly and aggressively, but despite your efforts to move the weight along, it doesn't move very fast.
- When you get to around rep number 8, this is where the real work kicks in.
- You pause at the top of the rep and take a deep breath, bring the weight down, and push it up again. It will take a great effort to get it back up.
- You will need to take one or two breaths before attempting the next rep because you know it's going to be difficult but not impossible.
- So take a few more breaths, bring the weight down, and drive up rep number 10.
- You now are wondering if you are able to get 11 and 12, but you have to attempt them because these are the reps that will give you the time and response you are looking for. With great effort you get through reps 11 and 12.

Great job!

If you were to time this set, you would find that it took between 40 and 70 seconds to complete (I have timed these sets thousands of times). Go through the list of exercises below and find out what your "challenging" 12 rep set is on each. Start out light on each exercise and always use good form. My most important rule is to always remember to breathe. Never hold your breath, especially during those last few difficult reps, as it can raise your blood pressure and be very dangerous.

These first three workouts are to find your challenging 12 rep max weight on each exercise. It will take a little time for each session to go through all the exercises until you get to that max set we are looking for, so put aside an hour for these workouts. Once you have the information, your workouts will all be less than 15 minutes!

Exercise List:
Workout One

- Leg Press, one leg at a time
- Smith Machine Squats
- Leg Extension
- Leg Curl
- Smith Machine Deadlift

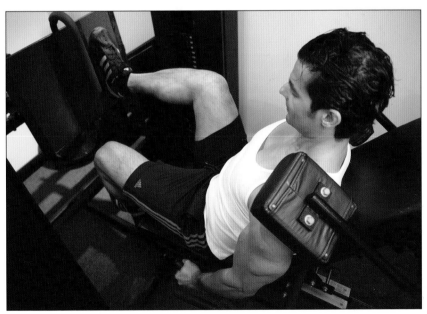

Leg Press One Leg at a Time—Right Leg Start

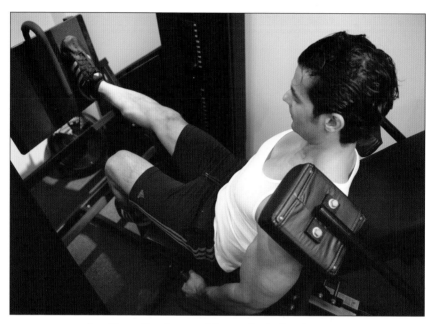

Leg Press One Leg at a Time—Right Leg Lockout

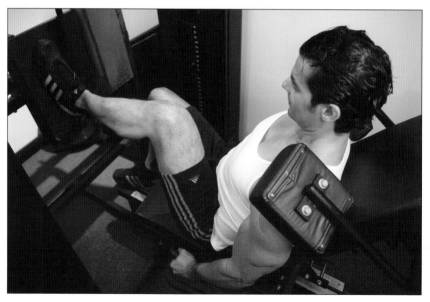

Leg Press One Leg at a Time—Left Leg Start

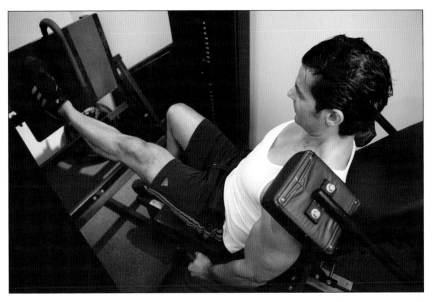

Leg Press One Leg at a Time—Left Leg Lockout

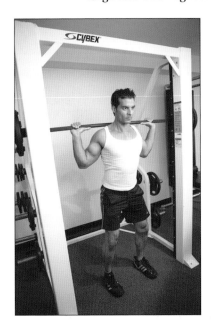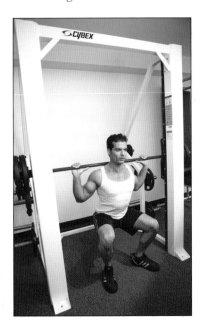

Smith Machine Squats

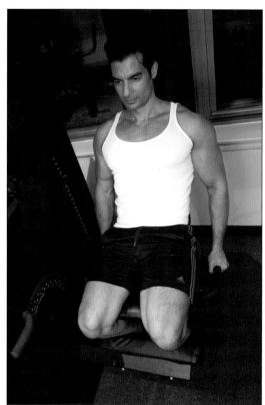

Leg Extension

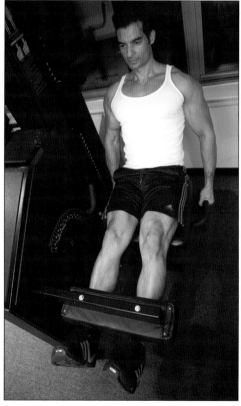

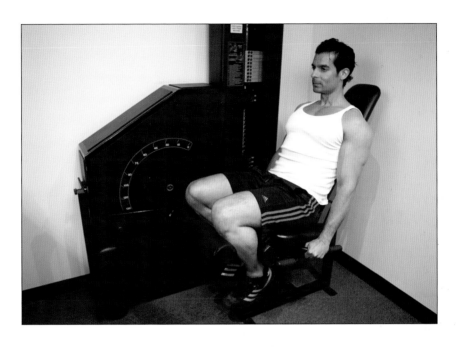

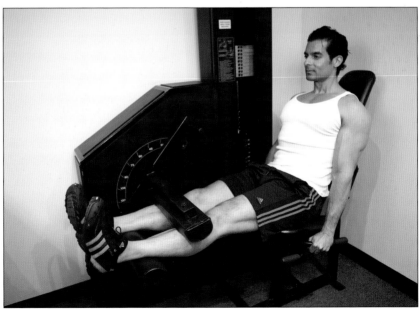

Seated Leg Curl

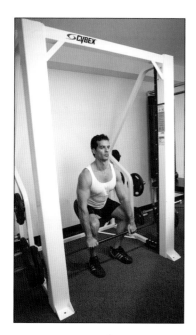 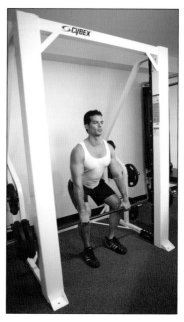

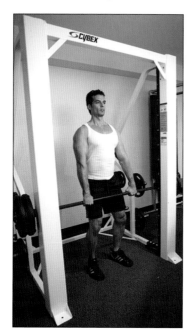

Smith Machine Deadlifts: Bottom, Midpoint, Lockout

Workout Two

- Chest Press
- One Arm Pushdowns
- Laterals
- Shoulder Press
- Close Grip Smith Machine Press
- Dip Machine

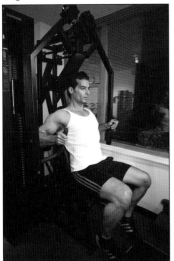
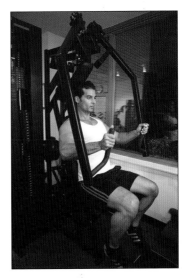

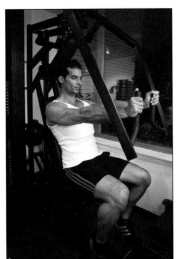

Workout Two: Chest Press—Start, Midpoint, Lockout

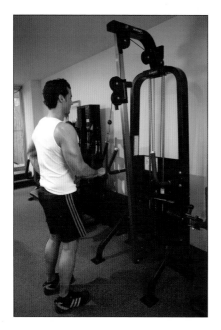
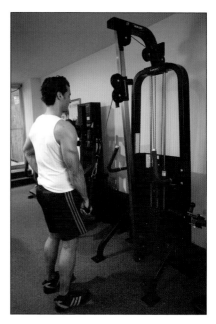

One Arm Pushdowns—Right Arm Start, Right Arm Lockout

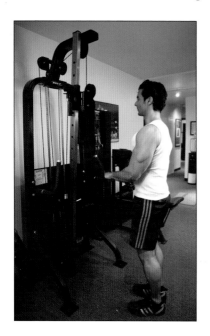
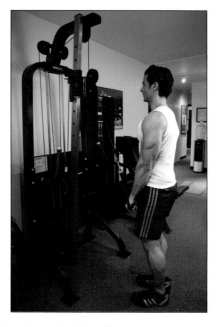

One Arm Pushdowns—Left Arm Start, Left Arm Lockout

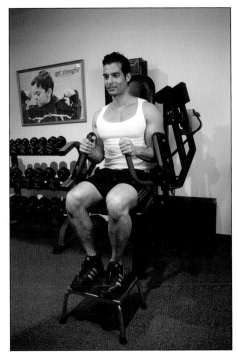

Lateral Raise Machine

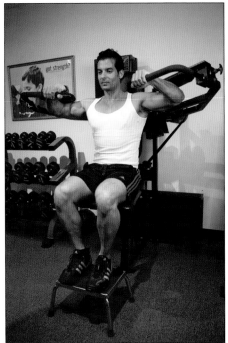

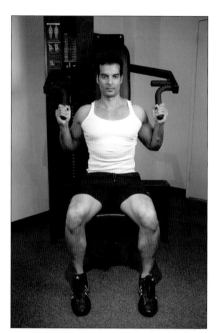

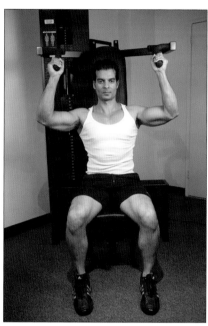

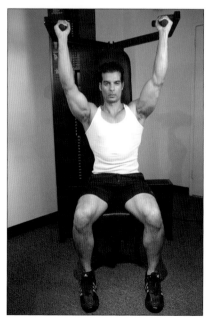

Shoulder Press

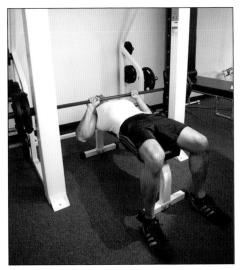

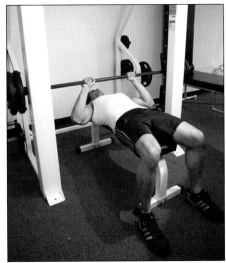

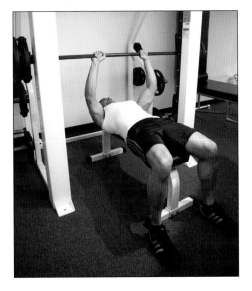

Close Grip Smith
Machine Bench Press

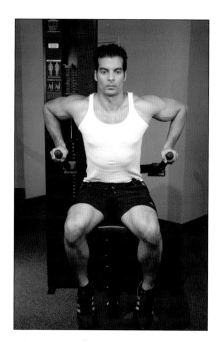

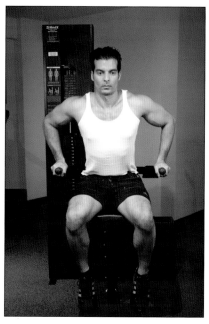

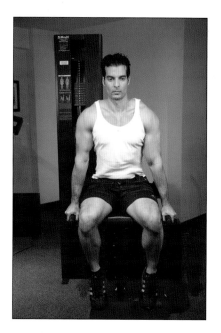

Dip Machine

Workout Three

- Straight Arm Pulldown
- Underhand Grip Pulldown
- Machine Curl
- Row Machine
- One Arm Cable Curl

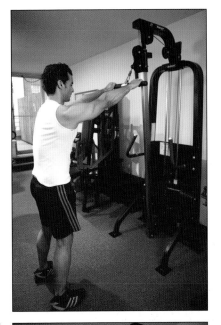

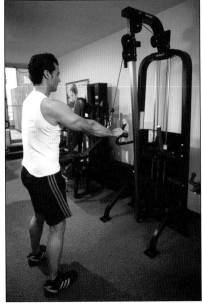

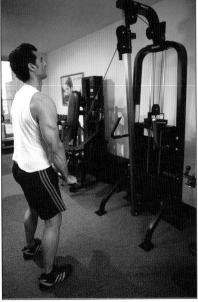

Straight Arm Pulldown

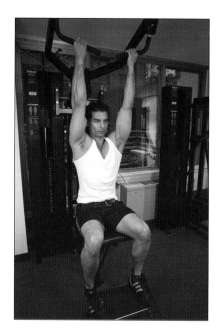
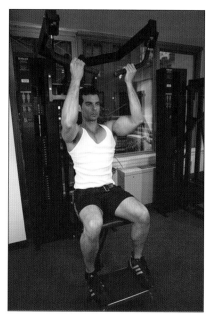
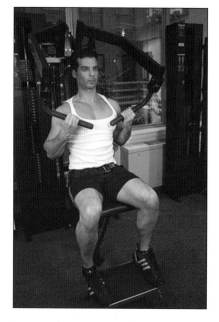

Underhand Grip Pulldown

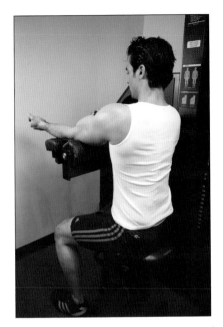
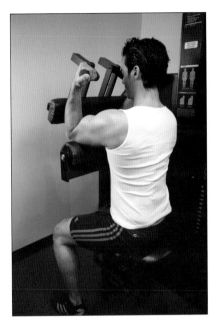

Machine Curl

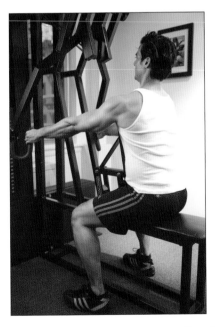
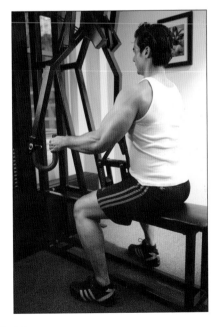

Row Machine

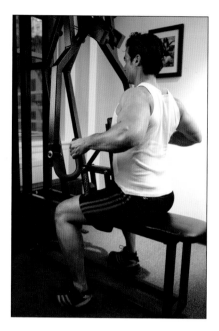

Row Machine

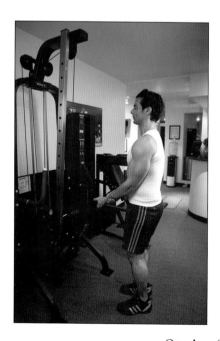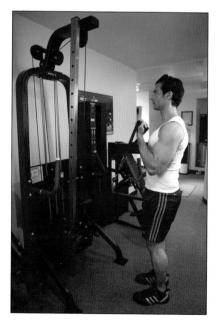

One Arm Cable Curl

Do the exercises listed for each workout on non-consecutive days. Take your time and do a few warm up sets on your way up to finding your 12 rep challenge set. Make sure to record your results. You can't change your body effectively without the proper information, so write everything down. The information you gather here is very important for the workouts that come later in the book. Keep in mind that these first three workouts are basically a "fact finding mission," and will take more time to get through than our High Intensity workouts will.

CHAPTER FOUR: HIGH INTENSITY HOME WORKOUTS

The High Intensity Home workouts will serve two purposes. It will be for those with no desire to go to the gym and act as a backup workout for those who travel.

My favorite High Intensity technique for home workouts is static contractions. "Statics," as we refer to them, involve no movement. You simply get into position and hold still. I've had many people over the years comment on the effectiveness of these exercises. Research shows that both men and women can gain up to 50 percent more strength and endurance using static contractions in less than 10 weeks.

So what are you waiting for? Hurry up and "don't move!"

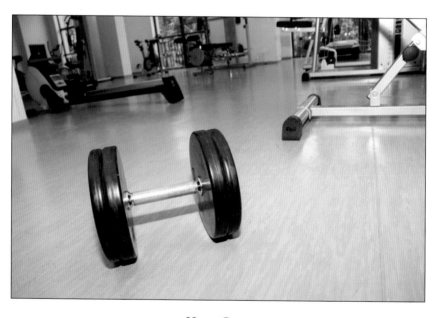

Home Gym

Home Workout Level One: Bodyweight Exercises

Equipment Needed: A wall and a floor

Number of Exercises: 3

Total Workout Time: 6 minutes

Bodyparts Worked: Total Body

Frequency: 3-5 times per week

1. Single Leg Wall Sit

Muscles Worked: Legs

High Intensity Method: Static Contractions

The Set: 60 seconds for each leg for a total of 120 seconds

Description: Do the exercises in the order listed with as little rest as possible.

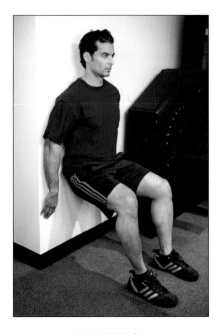

Basic Wall Sit

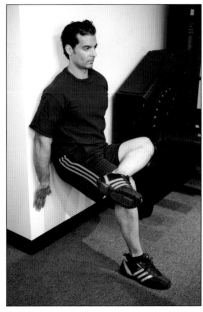

Left leg crossed. Try to hold this position for 60 seconds.

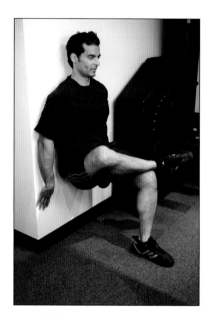

Right leg crossed. Your goal is 60 seconds on this side as well.

Start by getting into the wall sit position, then cross one leg up over your knee and hold. Your goal is 60 seconds for each side. If you can't hold the position for 60 seconds on each side, write it down on your workout chart and try to break the record next time. If this exercise is too difficult for you, try the standard two leg wall sit. When you get to 90 seconds on the two leg wall sit, advance to the single leg version.

2. Alternate Leg Raise Plank

Muscles Worked: Chest, Shoulders, Triceps, Abs, Lower Back, Glutes, and Hamstrings

High Intensity Method:

Static Contractions

The Set: Six 10-second static holds on each side for a total set time of 120 seconds

Description: Get into the plank position (the top part of a pushup)

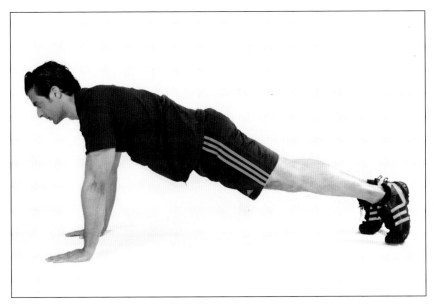

Basic Plank Position

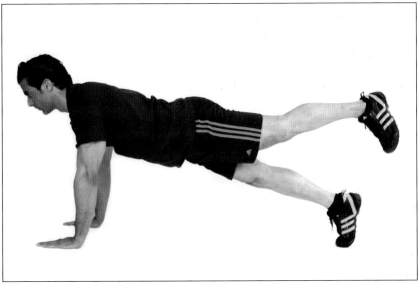

Left leg raised, hold for 10 seconds then switch to the right leg.

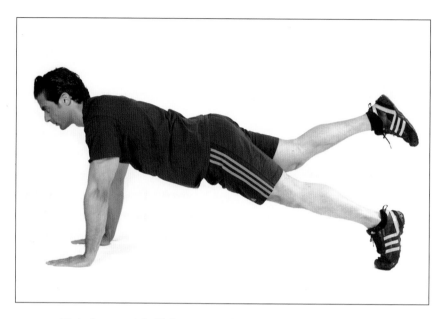

Right leg raised, hold for 10 seconds. Repeat 6 times on each side.

Raise one leg as shown and hold for 10 seconds, then switch sides to raise and hold the other leg for 10 seconds. Alternate for a total of 6 reps per side.

3. Alternate Arm Raise X-Plank

Muscles Worked: Chest, Shoulders, Triceps, Abs, Lower Back, Glutes, and Hamstrings

High Intensity Method: Static Contractions

The Set: 6-10 second static holds on each side for a total set time of 120 seconds

Description: Get into the wide X plank position (top part of a push up with wide leg stance)

The wide leg stance will give you the balance needed to raise one arm at a time.

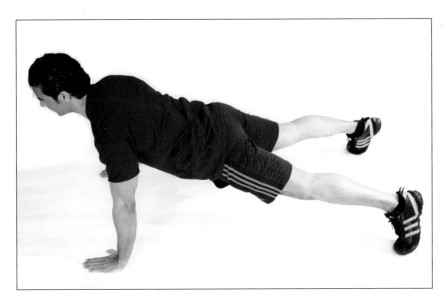

Basic X-Plank Position

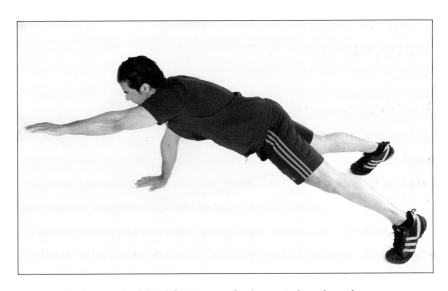

Left arm raised, hold for 10 seconds, then switch to the right arm.

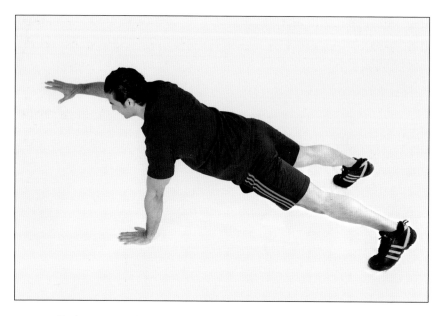

Right arm raised, hold for 10 seconds. Repeat 6 times on each side.

Raise one arm as shown below and hold for 10 seconds. Then switch sides to raise and hold the other arm as shown for 10 seconds. Alternate for a total of 6 reps per side.

Home Workout Level Two: High Intensity Dumbbell Routine with Cardio Kicker

Equipment Needed: Dumbbells, Treadmill, or Elliptical Machine (optional)

Number of Exercises: 9

Total Workout Time: 90 seconds

Bodyparts Worked: Total Body

Frequency: 3 times per week

At level two, we will kick it up a notch by adding dumbbells to the routine. Remember that anytime you increase the intensity of a workout, there must be a reduction in workout days to ensure adequate rest and recovery.

Start with a pair of 10 or 15 lb. dumbbells (and don't be afraid to trade up to the next highest pair when you master these). You will really feel the effectiveness of this workout when you get to the heavier dumbbells.

Do the exercises listed in order and with as little rest as possible.

Get into each position as shown and hold the contracted position for 10 seconds.

Start in a standing position with dumbbells at your sides:

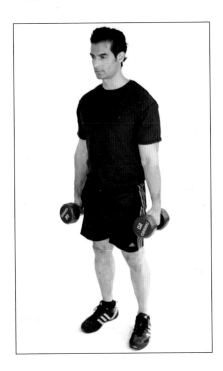

1. Lunge left
- Step forward with you left leg in the lunge position. Keep your back straight and hold for 10 seconds.

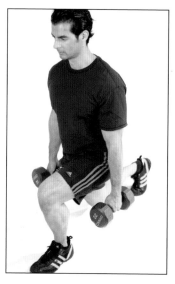

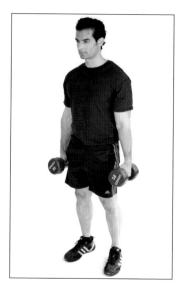

Left leg lunge. Hold the bottom position for 10 seconds. Don't let your knee touch the floor.

Back to the standing position

2. Lunge Right

- After the 10 second hold is completed with the left leg, return to the standing position and then step into the right leg lunge position for another 10 second hold.

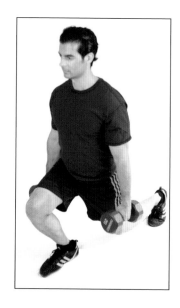

Right leg lunge. Hold the bottom position for 10 seconds. Don't let your knee touch the floor.

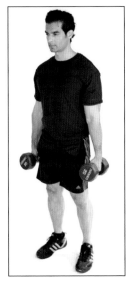

Back to the standing position

3. Plank

- Get into the plank position with dumbbells still in your hands and hold for 10 seconds.

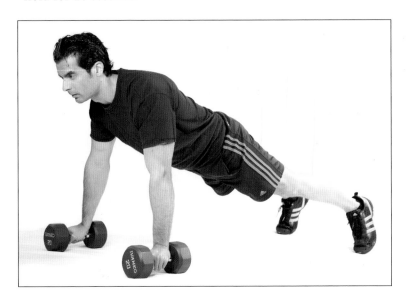

Get down into the plank position and hold for 10 seconds.

4. Plank – left leg up
- Raise your left leg and hold for the next 10 seconds

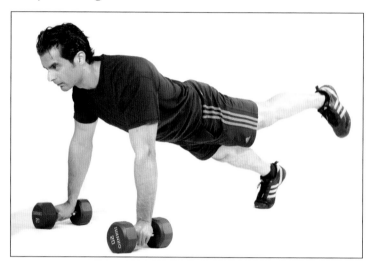

Left leg up and hold for 10 seconds

5. Plank – right leg up
- Switch to the right leg for 10 seconds

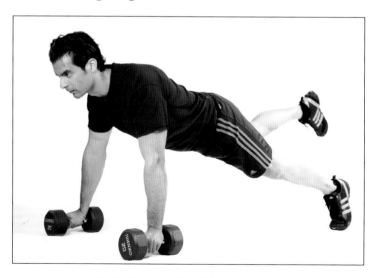

Right leg up and hold for 10 seconds

6. Plank Row – left arm up

- Widen your leg stance for better balance and raise your left arm up as shown for 10 seconds

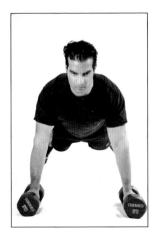

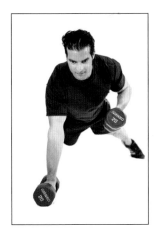

Plank Row starting position. Widen your leg stance for better balance.

Pull your left arm up as high as you can and hold for 10 seconds.

7. Plank Row – right arm up

- Switch to the right arm for 10 seconds

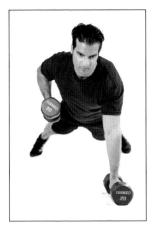

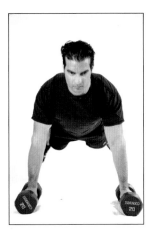

Plank Row right arm up. Again, pull up as high as you can and hold for 10 seconds.

Back to the Plank Row starting position then stand up with the dumbbells.

8. Biceps – 90 degrees

- After the Plank Rows are finished, get back into the standing position. Curl the weights up to 90 degrees and hold for 10 seconds.

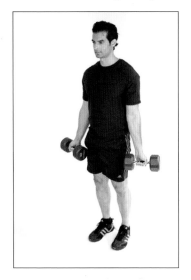 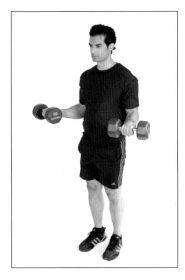

Back to the standing position and ready to do the biceps curl

Curl the dumbbells halfway up and hold for 10 seconds

9. Shoulder Press bottom position – transition

- After the bicep hold is complete continue to curl the weights up and rotate your hands to the neutral grip shoulder position as shown. This is a transition to the Shoulder press.

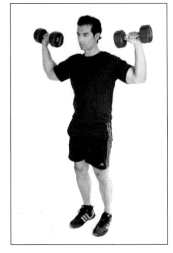

After your 10 second hold for biceps, finish curling the weight up to your shoulders and rotate into the bottom part of the Shoulder Press.

10. Shoulder Press

- Press the weights up to the top position of the shoulder press and hold for 10 seconds

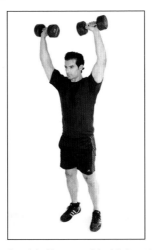

Press the dumbbells up and hold for 10 seconds

11. Shoulder Press bottom position – transition to finish

- Return to the bottom part of the shoulder press and slowly lower the weights to the floor as you are finished with the sequence.

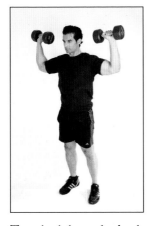 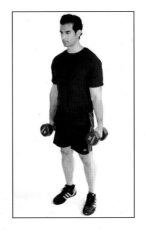

Then slowly lower the dumb-bells back down to the start of the Shoulder Press.

Finished!

High Intensity Cardio Kicker

Add one of these two options to your High Intensity Dumbbell Routine for increased metabolic stimulation. Don't get this confused with the boring cardio you've been told to do for years. This is "get your heart rate up, work hard, and be done with it" cardio!

Option One: High Intensity Power Walk

I know what you're thinking but power walking is an effective form of exercise. This is an option for those with no access to an elliptical machine. It is also the best option for those who are overweight and are just getting off the couch and into High Intensity workouts.

What I want you to do here is figure out a one-mile route. That may mean getting into your car and measuring off a mile or going to your local school track and finding out how many laps around it takes. Of course, if you live in New York City like I do, you know that 20 short blocks is the equivalent to one mile. Once you get your route laid out, get moving! The key here is to get the mile done as fast as possible. Figuring that if you walked on a treadmill at a 4 mile-per-hour pace, your one mile Power Walk should take around 15 minutes or less. Track your time and record your results. If you can beat your time by as much as a second, you are making progress. This can also

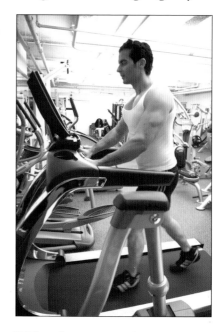

Walk as fast as you can for one mile. No jogging!

be done on a treadmill by walking as fast as you can until you reach one mile.

Option Two: High Intensity Elliptical Intervals

This is one of my favorites if you have access to one. Use the elliptical machine with the arm movement for best results. This will give you total body workout. Start by warming up. Level two for 5 minutes should be good, especially after the Dumbbell Routine. At the beginning of minute number 6, crank up the machine to the highest level. (That's level 15 on my machine but it varies from manufacturer to manufacturer.) Do the highest level for one minute and return to level two for a one minute rest. Alternate one minute each between levels 2 and 15 for a total of five minutes each, and then do a cool down on level 2 for five minutes until your heart rate is below 100. Make the most out of level 15 by really pushing and pulling those handles in conjunction with driving the foot pedals with your legs.

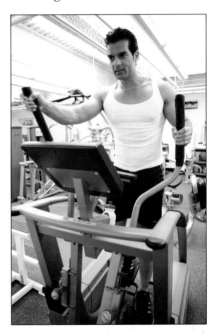

Keep in mind that the key to High Intensity Fitness is to work outside your comfort zone and push your workouts. This will keep your muscles from getting stale and resisting progress.

Get warmed up on the elliptical machine and then crank it up to the highest level for one minute then back down to level two for the next minute. Repeat five times so you get five High Intensity intervals for best results.

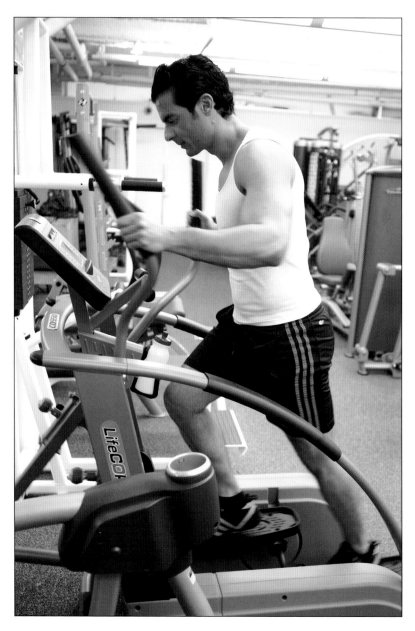

Really push hard with arms and legs for the High Intensity interval minutes.

CHAPTER FIVE:
HIGH INTENSITY LEGS

In this book I have set up three High Intensity workouts for you that will build and define your body with emphasis on the areas I know you want to target—abs, chest, and arms . . . but don't forget your legs. Working your legs really hard will actually help your overall look and stimulate your entire body. That's why I put this workout first. If possible, your workouts should be performed on non-consecutive days like Monday, Wednesday, Friday or Tuesday, Thursday, Saturday. This will give more rest and recovery time for your body. Each individual workout will be done only once per week to ensure maximum recovery of the body parts worked during each session. If you get into a jam schedule-wise and need to work out two days in a row or even three days in a row, go ahead and do it. It's more important not to skip your workouts, and since you won't be repeating the same workout until next week, you are still getting the maximum recovery time. This happens to my clients from time to time and sometimes you just have to make do. After looking at the exercises below, you may think I'm short-changing you, but this is all that you will have to do. Look, I can very easily lay out an exotic workout with 50 exercises that cover every different angle and option, but the truth of the matter is that our bodies (and muscles) aren't that complicated. One "big" basic exercise is better than 6 or 7 "small" exercises. What is a big or small exercise, you ask? A big exercise covers a large part of the body and involves many muscles. A small exercise is very specific and has little impact on stimulating your body.

Examples of big exercises are:

- Squats
- Leg Press
- Chest Press
- Pulldowns
- Dips and Pullups

Examples of "big" exercises are:

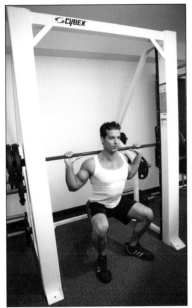

Squats

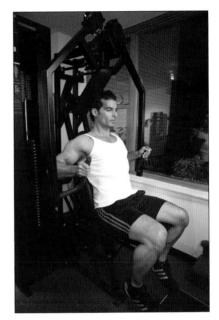

Chest Press

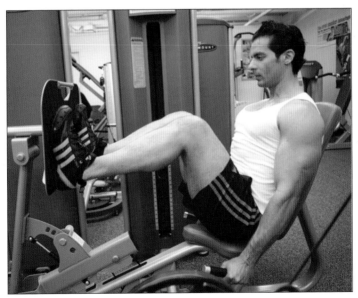

Leg Press

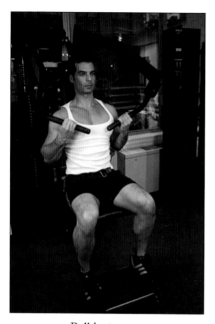

Pulldowns

Dips

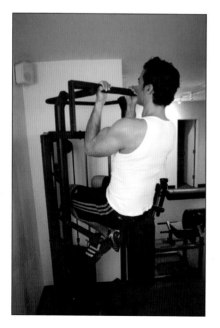

Pullups

SMALL EXERCISES INCLUDE:

- Flyes
- Laterals
- Curls
- Pushdowns
- Leg Extensions
- Leg Curls

Examples of "small" exercises are:

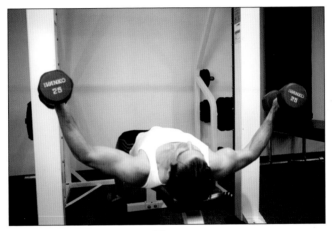

Flyes

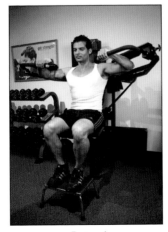

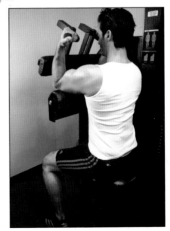

Laterals   Curls

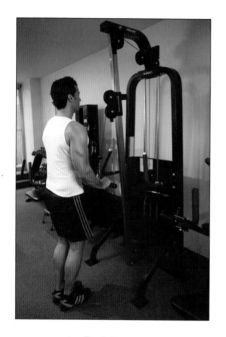

Pushdowns

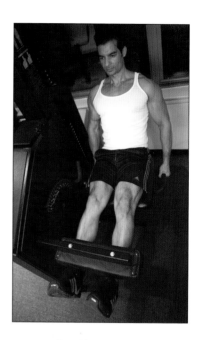

Leg Extensions

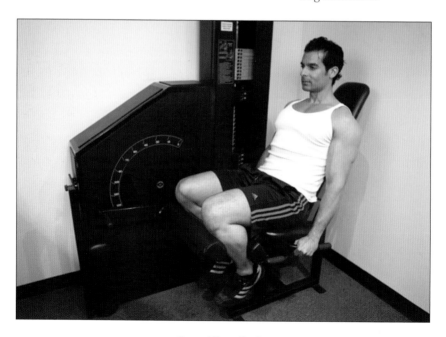

Seated Leg Curl

Now, it's not that I don't like any of these small exercises. They have great results when done properly, but emphasis should be placed on the big exercises. Don't worry, I will still show you how to use the small exercises to your advantage.

You are going to work your legs once a week and there will be three different versions of the workout to rotate through. Each workout will take less than 10 minutes if performed properly.

Leg Workout One, Week One

Warm up by getting on the elliptical machine or treadmill for 12 minutes. This is not a workout, but will serve as a warm-up for your legs by getting some blood flow to the area. If you don't feel like getting on the treadmill, just do two light warm-up sets of leg presses before you get to your working set.

Move from one exercise to the other in the order described with as little rest as possible between exercises. No warm-up sets are necessary during the workout.

1. Leg Press – 3 short, 1 long

After doing two warm-up sets, working up to your 12 rep max weight, you are ready to give this exercise your best effort for maximum results. We are going to emphasize the part of the leg press that is most effective and minimize the time spent on the part that has little or no effect. More specifically, the first few inches pushing forward is the most productive part of the leg press and the part where your legs are locked out straight does nothing for you.

- Get on the leg press machine.
- Choose your 12 rep max weight after your two warm-up sets (which don't count).
- Push the weight forward about 4-6 inches, and do that 3 times.
- On the 4th rep, push it all the way out. That series counts as ONE rep (3 short, 1 long).

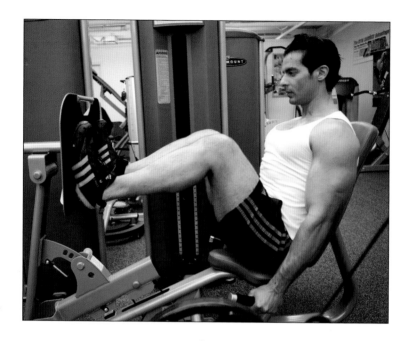

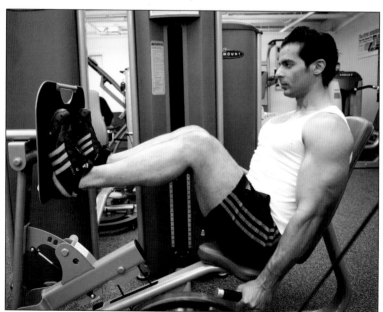

Just push halfway out for 3 reps and then lockout the 4th rep. That series counts as ONE rep.

- Go for a challenging set of 12 total "long" reps not counting the 3 short reps in between.

Remember that all you need is one set of each exercise, so give it your all!

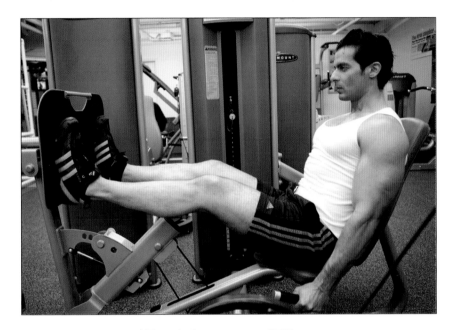

Every lockout counts as ONE rep

2. Leg press – 2 up, 1 down

Now we are going to emphasize the lowering portion of the leg press by pushing the weight up each time with two legs and lowering slowly with one. Working the muscles this way will ensure that you get deep into those stubborn leg fibers and stimulate muscle growth.

- Stay in the leg press machine and quickly reduce the weight by 50 percent.
- Push out with two feet.

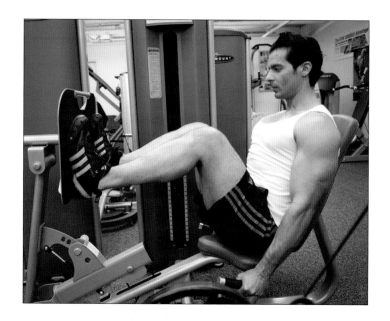

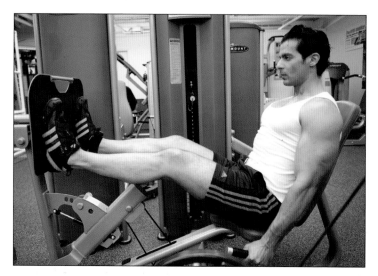

Push out with two legs

- Take your left foot off the foot plate and put it safely down and out of the way.

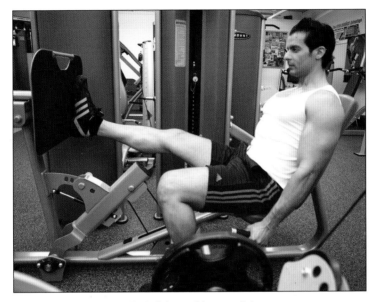

Drop the left leg safely out of the way

- Slowly lower the weight with only your right leg.

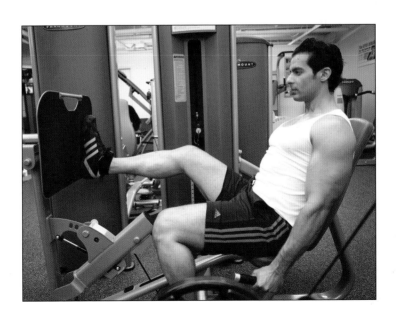

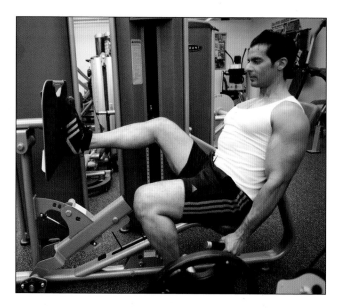

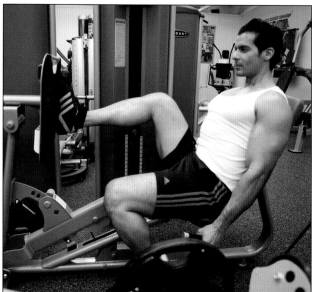

Slowly lower your right leg to the bottom. Try to take a full 4 seconds to do this.

- When you get to the bottom, push back up with two feet.

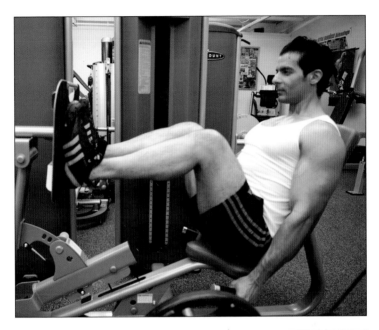

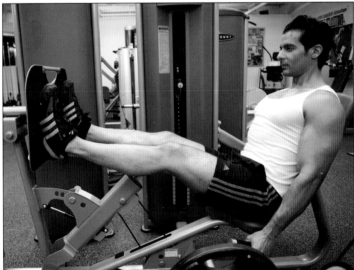

Put you left foot back up and push out with two legs

- This time, take your right foot off the foot plate and put it safely down and away.

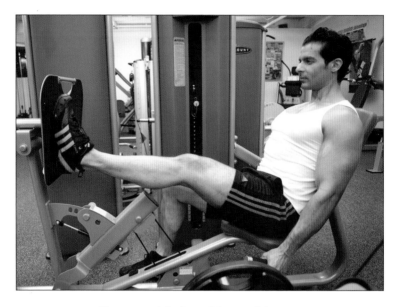

Drop your right leg safely out of the way

- Lower the weight with only your left leg as slow as possible. Make sure to never let the weight crash.

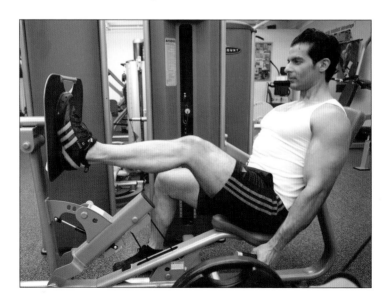

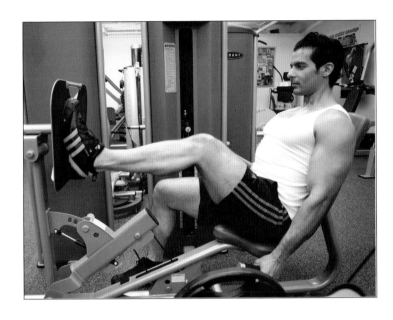

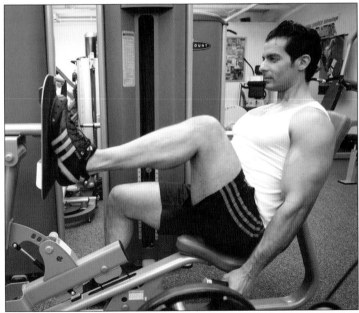

Slowly lower your left leg to the bottom. Try to take a full 4 seconds to do this.

- Do 6 reps with each leg. This is emphasizing the negative (or lowering) part of the exercise after you have exhausted the positive (or lifting) phase which will get deeper into the muscle fibers.

High Intensity Tip

Warning: You may be walking a little funny tomorrow night after doing the leg presses this way!

3. Single Leg Calf Raise

This is my favorite calf exercise. How many times do you see guys piling on an incredible amount of weight on the calf machine and then pumping out reps in a sloppy form? All that energy is wasted and they have nothing to show for it. This is not going to be you. The key to developing calves is not how much weight you lift, but how hard you contract and hold.

- Find a place to do your calf raises.
- Do one leg at a time and use the 5 second static hold technique at the top of each rep.
- 12 reps with each leg and you're done! Even though you can probably do more than 12 reps in this exercise, don't do them. Instead, concentrate on squeezing the top of each rep more intensely. Knowing that there is a limit in the number of reps will motivate you to work the exercise harder.

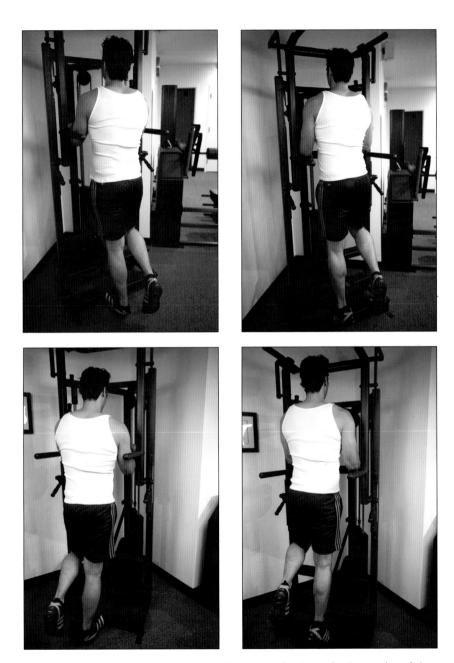

Do 12 reps with each leg. Squeeze and hold the top of each rep for 5 seconds and then get a good stretch before the next rep.

That's it—three exercises and you are done! All three exercises should add up to a total workout time of less than 10 minutes and the best part is you don't have to do it again until next week.

Leg Workout Two, Week Two

1. Smith Machine Squats

There's no special technique here. Do a warm-up set of 12 to 15 reps with 50 percent of your 12 rep max weight. Make sure to set the safeties so the bottom of the squat is at 90 degrees. The safeties will also serve as protection in case you can't get back up from a rep.

- Do your 12 rep max set.

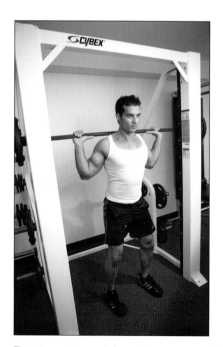 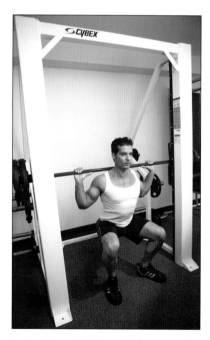

Do 12 reps in good form after warm up. Reps 9, 10, 11, and 12 should be a struggle.

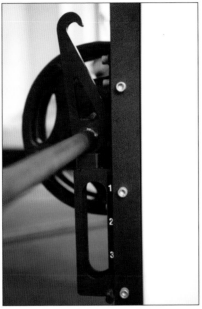

Set the safeties an inch below the bottom position of the squat where your thighs are parallel to the floor. This way, if you can't make it back up for one of the reps, you won't get hurt. Safety first!

2. Leg Extension – 2 up, 1 down

- Get into the leg extension machine according to your settings.
- Choose a weight that is 50 percent of your current 12 rep max.
- Slowly raise both legs up to full extension and hold at the top.
- Lower your left leg while the right leg holds the weight up.
- Now slowly lower your right leg (lowering your right leg counts as one rep).
- Raise both legs up again, but this time hold the weight with your left leg and drop your right leg down, then slowly lower your left leg back to the starting position.

Get the idea? Keep repeating this sequence until you get 6 reps with each leg.

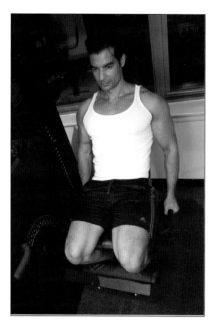 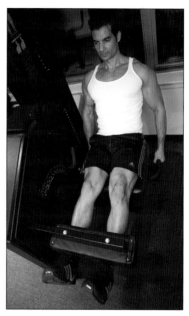

From the starting position, extend both legs up to the lockout position.

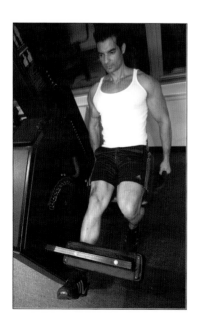

Lower your left leg and hold the weight with the right leg.

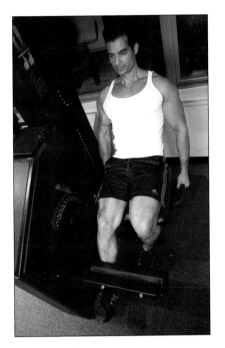

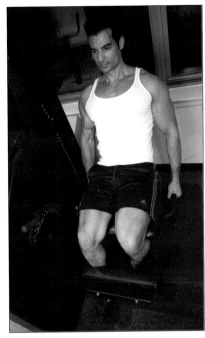

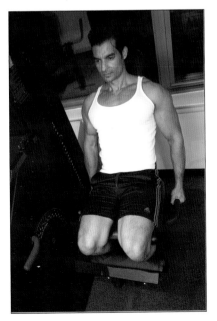

Slowly lower your right leg to the bottom. Try to take a full 4 seconds to do this.

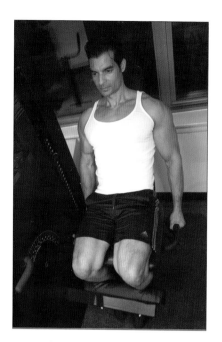

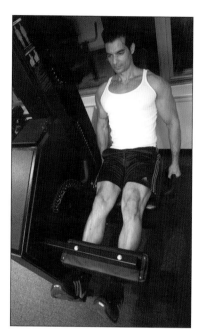

Extend both legs back up to the top position.

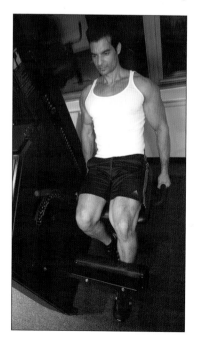

Slowly lower your left leg to the bottom. Try to take a full 4 seconds to do this. Repeat the sequence and do 6 reps with each leg.

3. Single Leg Calf Raise

- Find a place to do your calf raises
- Do one leg at a time and use the 5 second static hold technique at the top of each rep
- 12 reps with each leg and you're done! Even though you can probably do more than 12 reps in this exercise, don't do them. Instead, concentrate on squeezing the top of each reps more intensely. Knowing that there is a limit in the number of reps will motivate you to work the exercise harder.

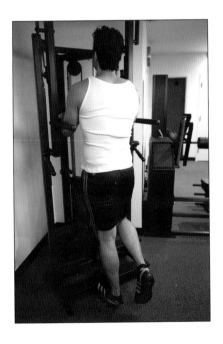 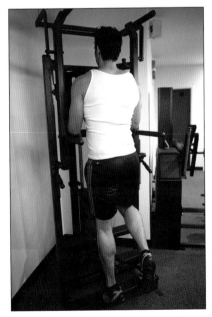

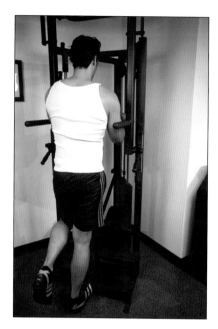 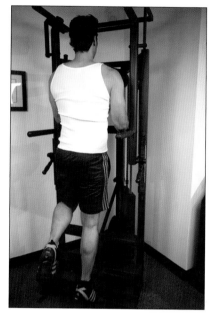

Do 12 reps with each leg. Squeeze and hold the top of each rep for 5 seconds and then get a good stretch before the next rep.

Leg Workout Three, Week Three

1. Leg Curl

- Do your 12 reps max set.
- Remember to start the first rep very slowly and then get more aggressive as you get into the set. Always use good form and remember to breathe throughout.

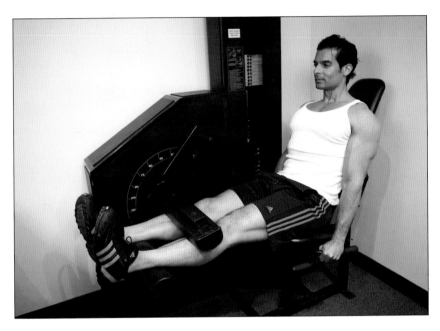

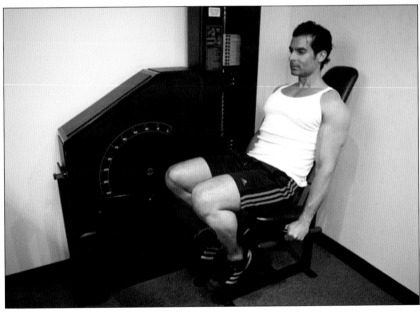

Seated Leg Curl: Start and finish

2. Smith Machine Deadlift

- Talk about a "big" exercise—this is one of the biggest. It will practically stimulate your whole body.
- We are shooting for our 12 rep max set here, nothing fancy.
- Get into the position shown and descend slowly into the first rep. This exercise is like doing a squat but with the weight in your hands and not on your back. Keep your back flat and look straight ahead for the best form. The last few reps should be a real challenge so give it your all!

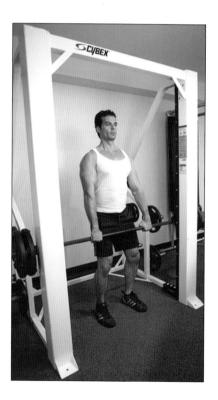 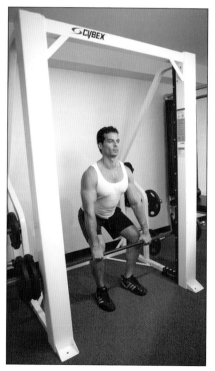

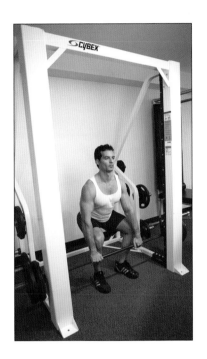

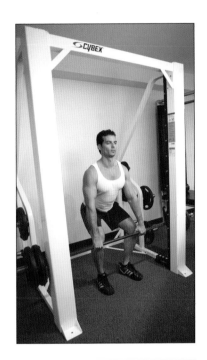

Smith Machine Deadlifts: Keep your back flat and your head up. The last few reps will require a few breaths at the top to get ready for the next attempt.

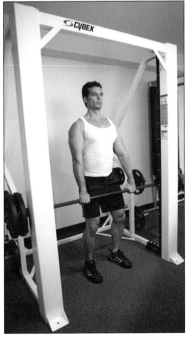

3. Single Leg Calf Raise

- Find a place to do your calf raises
- Do one leg at a time and use the 5 second static hold technique at the top of each rep
- Twelve reps with each leg and you're done! You heard me say it before, but squeeze those babies at the top of each rep fro 5 full seconds and get a good stretch at the bottom!

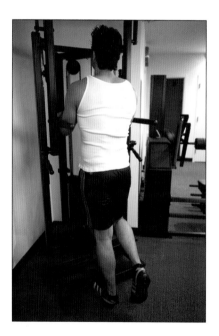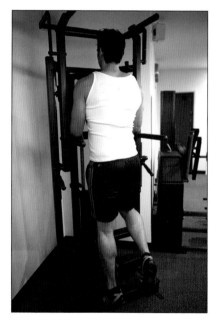

You know the drill here. Squeeze hard at the top and get 'em done!

CHAPTER SIX: HIGH INTENSITY PUSH

Now we are going to group all the "pushing" exercises together. I am arranging your workouts three parts: legs, push, and pull. By separating the body into three sections, it will ensure better recovery in between workouts and give you faster results. The pushing muscles are chest, shoulders, and triceps. I'm sure that most of you are interested in tightening up the back of your arms (triceps), so I will make sure there is a special high intensity technique for them.

Push Workout One, Week One

1. Flat Dumbbell Flies

We are going to use a stretch and hold technique to get the most out of this exercise. Remember that there is a compromise here. You will work harder, but you only have to do one set.

- Choose a weight that will allow 12 smooth reps (not a challenging 12 rep weight).
- Get on the bench with dumbbells positioned over your chest.
- Slowly (extra slow on the first rep) stretch out into the bottom position shown. Hold it there for 5 seconds and squeeze back up to the top in a controlled manner. 12 reps performed this way will get you 60-90 seconds of working time on these muscles and prepare you for the next exercise.
- If you feel the weight is becoming very doable, choose a heavier weight next time.

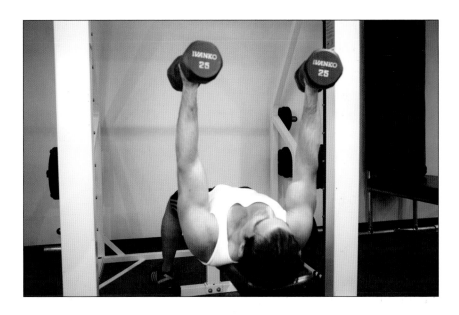

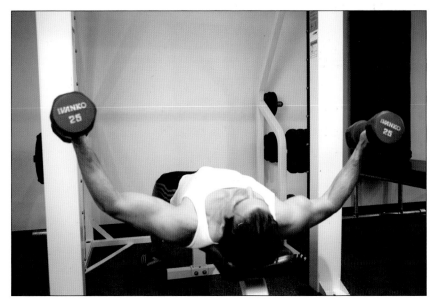

Flat Dumbbell Flies: Hold for a count of 5 in the stretched position. Slowly return to the top. You will feel your pecs working on every rep with this technique.

Pec Deck—Optional

An alternative to the dumbbell flies is the Pec Deck machine. You can switch off each workout with the dumbbell flies or stick with whichever one feels more comfortable.

- Get into the machine.
- Bring the handles to the fully contracted position and hold for 5 seconds.
- Repeat for 12 reps and add weight when the 12th rep becomes easy.

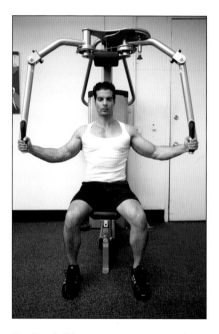 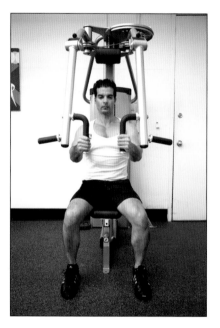

Pec Deck: This a great exercise to alternate the dumbbell flies with each workout. The flies emphasize the stretched position and the pec deck will work the contracted position.

2. Chest Press

- Get into the chest press machine and pump out your 12 rep max. You should need to take a few breaths one the last few reps at the lockout position before attempting the next rep, as the set is now becoming very challenging. If you are able to do all 12 reps smoothly and without any breaks during the set, you will need more weight next time . . . so crank it up!

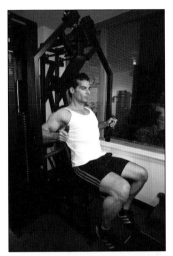 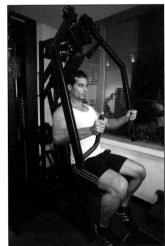

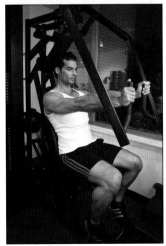

Chest Press: Start, Midpoint, Lockout

3. Two Arm Pushdowns

Let's finish off our Push workout with some direct triceps work. We will use this exercise as a warm-up for the Negative Only Dips. Set up the machine with a single cable handle.

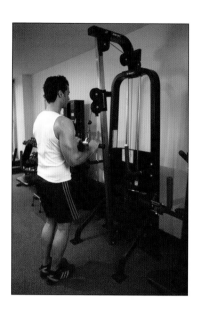

- You are already warmed up from your other "pushing" exercises, so just get to it and do a strong 12 rep max set. Use good form on all reps—even when the weight seems immovable.

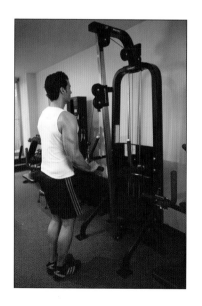
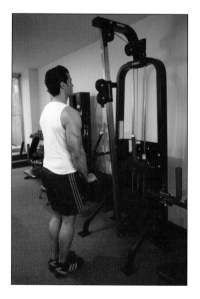

Two Arm Pushdowns: Start, Midpoint, Lockout

4. Negative Only Dips

Make sure to only do the lowering part of this exercise and limit yourself to THREE reps!

- Climb up into position and lower yourself as slowly as possible. As soon as you get to the bottom, put your feet down and climb right back up for the next rep. Your goal is to get 40-70 seconds worth of "lowering" time in the three reps. Use a stopwatch to keep track. The pushdown set you do before this will always keep this exercise challenging.

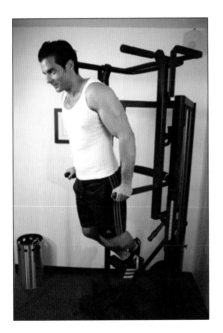 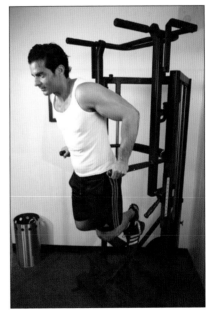

Negative Only Dips: Climb into position and lower yourself as slowly as possible. Three reps is all it takes to get the job done.

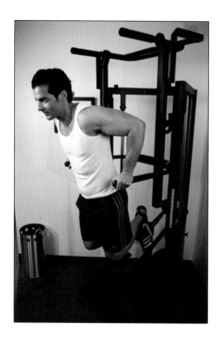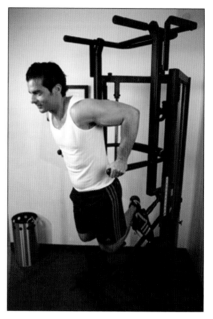

Some of my clients can lower themselves as slowly as 30 seconds for each of the 3 reps. When this happens, we add additional weight to the next workout.

Four exercises and the High Intensity Push Workout is finished. Here are the Push workouts you will use next week and the week after.

Push Workout Two, Week Two

In week two, we will emphasize shoulders and triceps in our Push workout. Not only are these workouts time efficient and intense, but the exercise variations will develop a balanced look.

1. Laterals

The lateral machine is going to isolate the side delts of your shoulders. This will pre-exhaust the muscles for the big exercise to follow (shoulder press) and make it much more effective.

- Get set up in your Lateral Raise machine.
- Raise the weight to a point just above parallel to the floor.
- Use the 5 second static technique at the top of each rep.
- Use a weight that will challenge you for 12 reps.

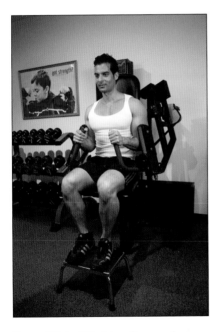 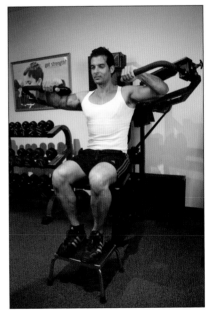

Lateral Raise Machine: Start at the top position. Hold the top position for a full 5 seconds before lowering. This would be an unreasonable request if you were doing many sets of the same exercise, so since you are only doing one, make sure to give it your all!

2. Shoulder Press

- Get to the shoulder press machine as soon as possible after doing your lat raises to get the most out of this combination.
- Use the "neutral grip" option, which is where the palms of your hands are facing each other when you grab the handles.
- Bang out 12 of these babies and make sure that reps 9, 10, 11, and 12 are a struggle.

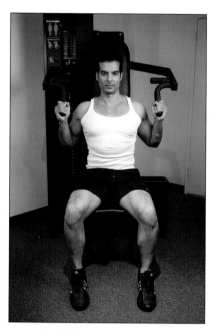

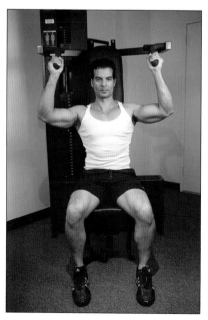

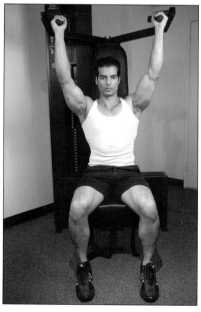

Shoulder Press: Start, Midpoint, and Lockout. Your shoulders are already fatigued from the lat raises, so you will get much more from this exercise now.

3. Close Grip Smith Machine Press

This exercise will tie the whole workout together. It's a great movement for all the pushing muscles (chest, shoulders, and triceps).

- Set up the Smith Machine with a flat bench.
- Set the safeties so that the bar will not touch your chest and instead stop about 1-2" above.

Since there is more muscle activation at the bottom of this movement than in the lockout position, we will use the 3 short, 1 long method to emphasize the lower, more intense portion of the exercise.

- Lower the first rep very slowly.
- Barely touch the safeties. Never bounce or bang into them.
- Push halfway up for 3 short reps and then lock out the 4th.

That whole sequence counts as ONE rep: 3 short & 1 long = one.

- Do a 12 rep max set.

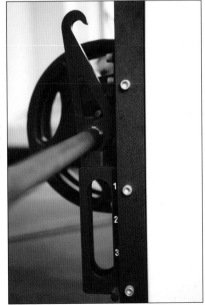

Here is a close-up shot of the safeties. Set them so the bar touches down a few inches above your chest. Never bounce off them.

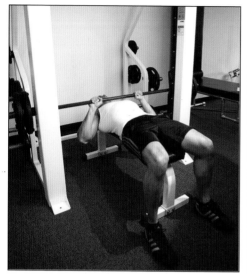 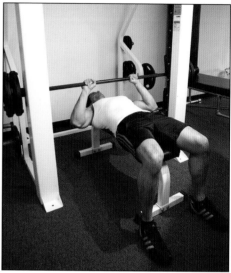

Push up halfway for 3 reps and then lock out the 4th—that sequence counts as ONE rep.

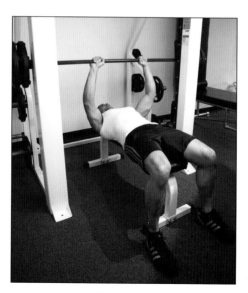

The lockout

Push Workout Three, Week Three

Okay, let's stop playing around and get to some serious work! The last two push workouts are very tough and effective, but I have saved the most intense for last. This workout consists of just one exercise that will exploit all of the different ways to get deep into the muscle fibers. Positive, Static, and Negative strength.

1. Dips or Dip Machine

If you are strong enough to do a set of dips, then just jump up there and go right ahead. Your goal is 12 reps while lowering yourself to the 90 degree arm position. If you are able to get to 12 reps easily, your next step is to lower yourself slowly over 4 seconds and push up more aggressively. If slowing down your reps becomes doable, then it's time to add weight. That can be accomplished with a weight belt that will allow you to hang a dumbbell or a plate.

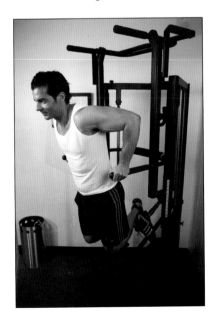 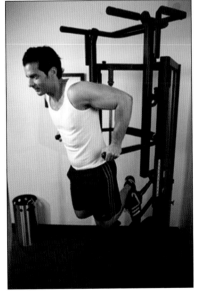

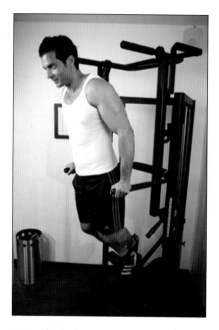 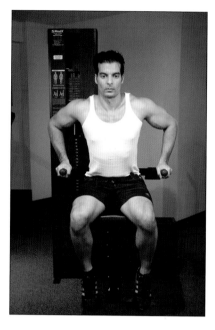

Dips: If you can do 12 reps in good form, then try slowing the rep speed down and making the 12 reps last for 40 to 70 seconds. This can be done by lowering each rep with a count of 4 and pushing up in 2. Add weight if you can do 12 reps in 70 seconds or more.

Dip Machine: Use this option if you are unable to do dips with your bodyweight. Keep increasing your strength with this exercise as your goal is to be able to do bodyweight dips.

If you are unable to do Dips with your bodyweight, then find its equivalent in the gym. Every gym these days has either a machine that will assist you with chins and dips or an individual dip machine. Whichever you choose, do a 12 rep max set then go immediately to a set of dip bars so you can do the next version of our High Intensity Dip workout.

2. Static Dips

- Get into the top part of this exercise.
- Bend your elbows slightly and hold that position for up to 30 seconds. You can time yourself with a watch, stopwatch, or cell phone. After you complete the 30 second hold, step down and take a short break before doing the last version of this exercise.

3. Negative Only Dips

- Getting back up on the same dips bars into the top position, you will lower yourself as

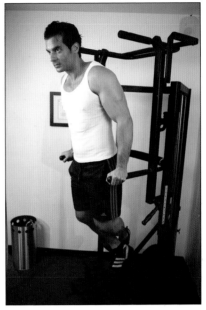

After your set of dips or dip machine, get into position on the dips bars, bend your elbows slightly, and hold for up to 30 seconds. You will be adding weight to this exercise very soon!

slowly as possible for three reps total with your goal being a minimum of 40 seconds and a maximum of 60 seconds in three reps.

- After you lower yourself for the first rep, put your feet on the floor, take a deep breath, and climb back up into the top position. Again lower yourself as slowly as possible and try to accumulate as many seconds as you can.
- Do the third rep the same way. You will most likely notice that you achieved the most time on the first rep, a little less on the second, and much less on the third. That's a good thing! It means that you were stimulating the muscles effectively.
- Record your progress and start the push cycle over again next week.

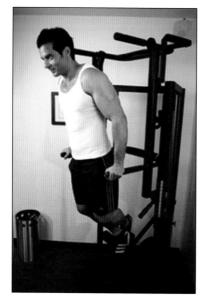
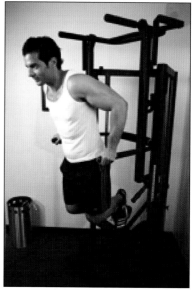
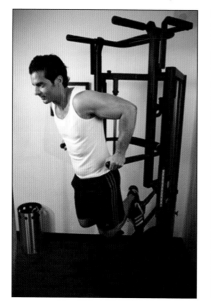
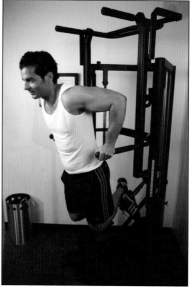

No lifting here, only lowering. Climb up and get into position. Lower yourself as slowly as possible. You want to accumulate as many seconds as you can in three "lowering only" reps. If you can do three 30 second reps, then it's time to add weight.

CHAPTER SEVEN:
HIGH INTENSITY PULL

The "pulling" muscles are basically the muscles of the back and biceps, but with my High Intensity workouts, a few more muscles usually get involved. A strong back will give you that "V" shape you're looking for and it's the big pulling exercises like underhand grip chins that take your biceps to the next level.

Pull Workout One, Week One

This first workout will emphasize the muscles of the upper back. We will pre-exhaust the back muscles with two exercises and then finish off the biceps, which will already be fatigued from the pulldown exercise.

1. Straight Arm Pulldown

This exercise is much better than doing pullovers with a dumbbell because there is tension on the muscles at the bottom of the exercise where with the dumbbell pullover there is none.

- Stand in front of a cable machine that has a short, straight bar attached.
- Grip the handles and take two steps back.
- From a fully stretched position with arms only slightly bent, bring your hands down to your thighs.
- Use the 5 second hold technique to increase the effectiveness of the movement.
- Do a 12 rep max on this set and get over to the pulldown machine ASAP.

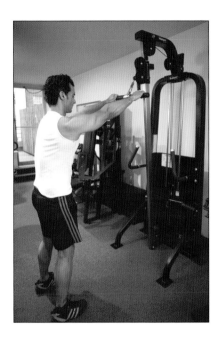

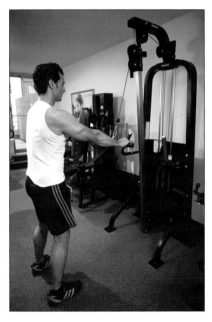

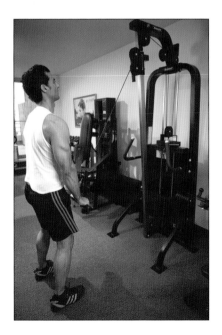

Straight Arm Pulldown: Start, Mid-point, Finish

2. Underhand Grip Pulldown

- Select the weight that will challenge you for 12 reps.
- Use a shoulder width underhand grip.
- Get into position with arms stretched.
- Pull down slowly on the first rep, holding at the bottom for a count of 5 and then back up. Get more aggressive with each rep but make sure you hold for a count of 5 at the bottom.
- Keep your back flat by sitting up straight throughout the set and remember to breathe even when the reps get tough.

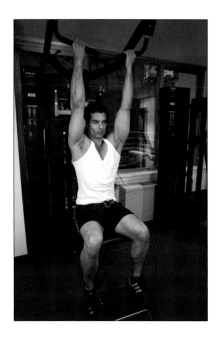 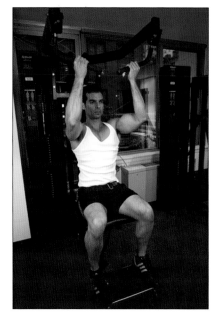

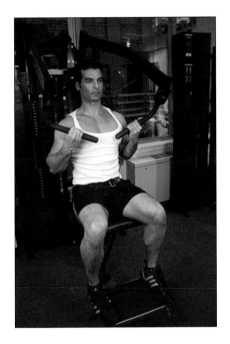

Underhand Grip Pulldown: The 5 second hold at the bottom of each rep will ensure that you spend an adequate amount of time stimulating the working muscles.

3. Machine Curl

- The machine curl will isolate the biceps better than a dumbbell or barbell. It will also encourage better form when the set gets difficult.
- Do a 12 rep max set here and use the 5 second hold technique in the contracted position.
- Three sets and you are done, so make them count!

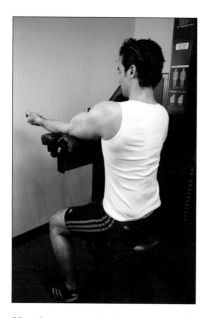 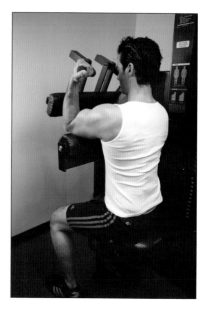

Your biceps are already pre-fatigued from the Underhand Grip Pulldowns. One set using the 5 second hold technique in the contracted position will be all you'll need to work your biceps thoroughly.

Pull Workout Two, Week Two

I'm giving you the most intense workout of the Pull cycle in week two. Why? Better to get this over with sooner rather than later. This is going to be like the Dip exercise was in the Push workout so you will recognize the workout right away.

1. Underhand Grip Chins or Pulldowns

The day that you can do an underhand chin-up on your own will be the single most rewarding accomplishment in your workouts.

- Option One: Hang from a chin-up bar with an underhand grip and pull yourself up until your chin gets over the bar for as many reps as you can. If you can do one rep this time, then your goal will be two reps next time. If you can't do any chin-ups, go straight to option two.

- Option Two: Using the chin assisst machine, select a weight that assists you only enough to get through 8 reps easily so that you'll have to fight for the last 4.
- Option Three: Do a 12 rep max set on the underhand grip pulldown bar, but try to increase the weight as often as possible to become strong enough to attempt chin-ups.

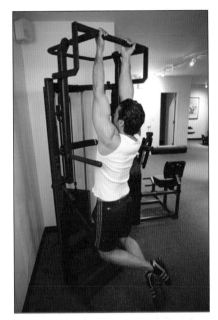

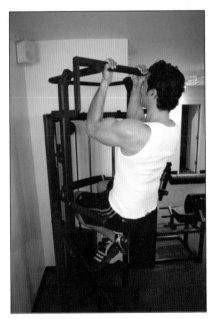

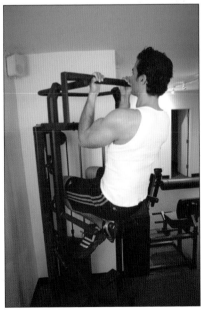

Chin-ups rule! Anytime I see people in the gym who are good at chin-ups they are always in great shape. A lean body with a "V" shape and great arms is the way to go . . . and chin-ups will get you there.

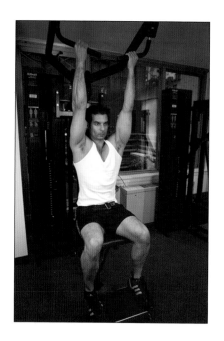 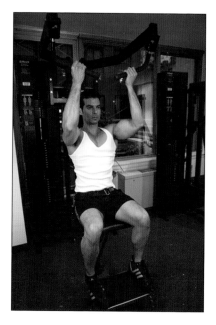

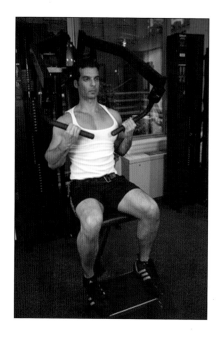

Use Underhand Grip Pulldowns to increase your strength until you are strong enough for chin-ups.

2. Static Hold Chin-ups

Even if you can't do a single chin-up, you will be able to hold the top position for some time.

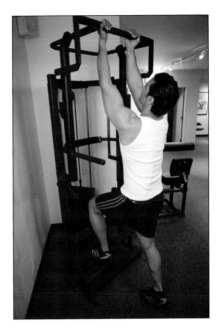

- Climb up into the top position of the chin-up and attempt to hold for 30 seconds.
- Keep your knees up at a 90 degree position so you can work your abs as well.
- Lower yourself carefully after you reach 30 seconds or can't hold anymore.

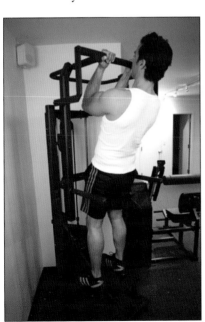

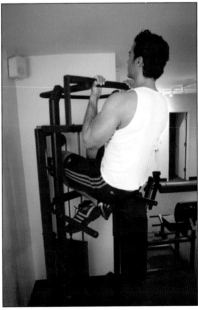

Step up into position and hold. Slowly lower yourself to the fully stretched position when you can't hold anymore or reach 30 seconds.

3. Negative Only Chin-ups

Now that you have weakened your muscles positively (the lifting phase) and statically (the holding phase), we are going to finish them off with a negative only strength exercise, which means that all you have to do is lower the weight (or yourself). No lifting.

- For this set of underhand grip chins, only 3 reps are required.
- Climb up to the top position and hold yourself statically just like in the last set. This time, only hold for 5 seconds and then start to lower yourself, again keeping your knees up to work your abs.
- Go as slowly as possible. I mean really fight it all the way down. When you reach the fully stretched position at the bottom, put your feet down rest for a second and check your time.

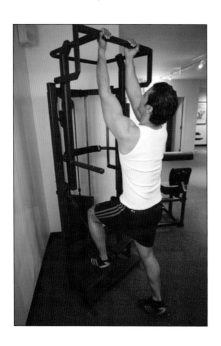 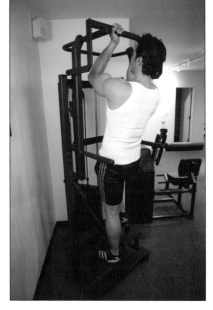

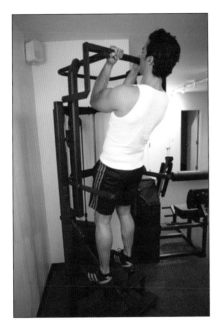
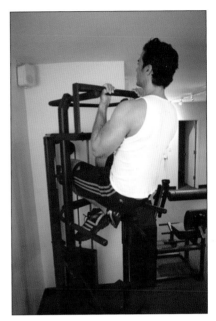

Climb up into position and hold for only a second before lowering.

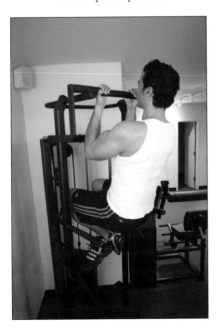
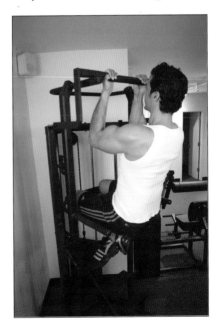

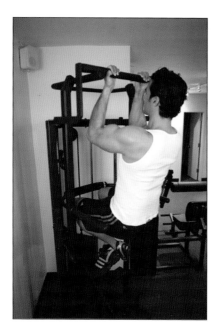

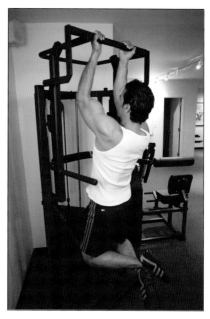

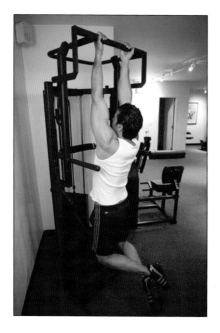

Lower as slowly as possible with your goal being 3 negative only reps lasting 30 seconds each.

How many seconds did it take you to hold and lower? Make a quick note of it and then climb back up and do it again.

Your goal is to be able to do three negative only reps for 30 seconds each. No matter how strong you get, this workout will always be a challenge and deliver results.

Pull Workout Three, Week Three

Workout Three of this cycle is a little less intense than last week's workout but no less effective. We will be targeting the mid-back, rear delts (back of the shoulders), and biceps in a different way. The great thing about all of these High Intensity workouts is that your body will never get accustomed to any one workout and the variety will keep you mentally motivated.

1. Underhand Grip Bodyweight Row

- Use the Smith Machine for this exercise. Get into the position shown where you are hanging by your arms with an underhand grip. We are using the underhand grip for all these pulling exercises because it is the strongest grip out of all the options and will give you the greatest and fastest results. Make sure your hips are up and your legs are at a 90 degree position to start.
- Pull yourself up to the bar or as high as you can go. Try to arch your back a little as you go up. This will increase the contraction of the mid-back muscles.
- Aim for 12 reps. If you are able to get 12 reps with no problem, feel free to torture yourself more by holding the top position for 5 seconds which will ensure that you get the appropriate amount of time on the exercise. Remember that if you were working with me at my gym, I would probably make you hold it a little longer.

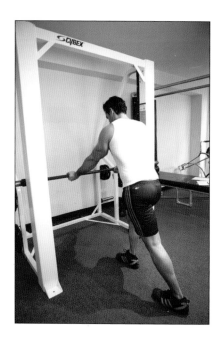
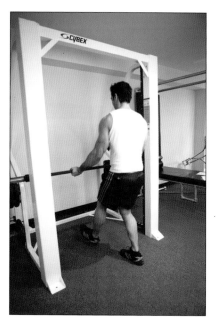
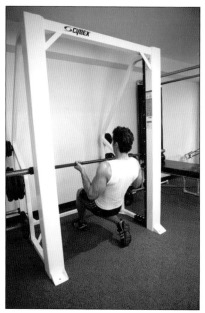
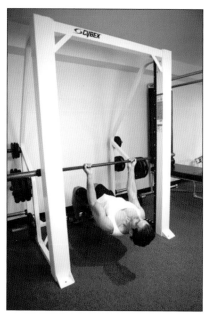

Set the bar about waist high. Use an underhand grip and walk under the bar to get into position. Starting position is arms hanging with a flat back.

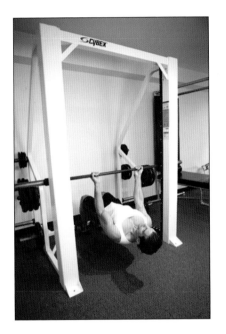

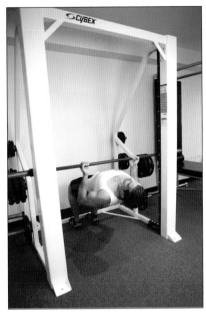

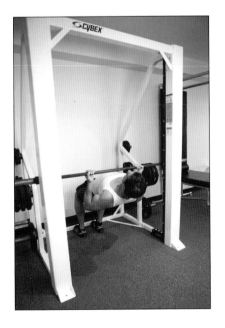

Pull up until your chest touches the bar. Use the "squeeze and hold" technique in the top contracted position. One set is all you need.

2. Row Machine

This exercise is similar to what we just did, but we are going to opt for the neutral grip handles to be different from the last exercise. The neutral grip is where the palms of your hands are facing each other.

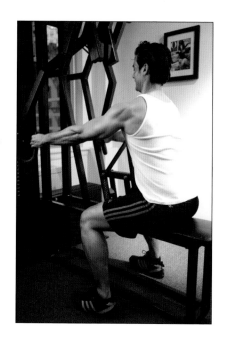

- Same deal here. Do your 12 rep max with 5 second holds at the top.

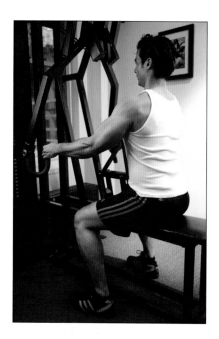

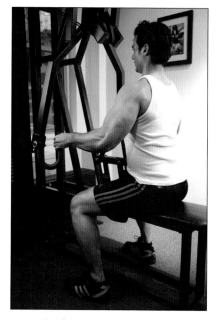

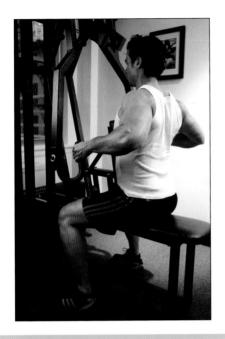

Row Machine: Pull back and hold for 5 seconds in the contracted position.

High Intensity Tip

Remember to use good form at all times. Do not swing the weight up when it becomes difficult, as it can result in a lower back injury.

3. One Arm Cable Curl

This exercise is really cool and will carve out some major detail in your biceps.

- Stand in front of the cable machine with a single handle cable attachment. Select a weight that is 10 lbs. heavier than your 12 rep max.
- Since the weight is 10 lbs. heavier than your 12 rep max, your reps should fall short of 12. Let's say that you start to fail around rep 8. Assist yourself with your free hand and use both to pull the weight up into position. Then lower slowly with one arm until you finish the remaining reps to make 12.

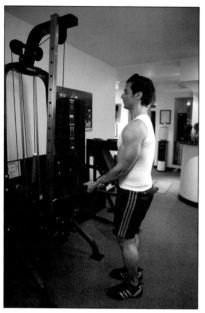

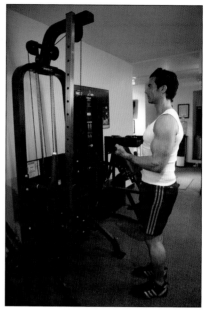

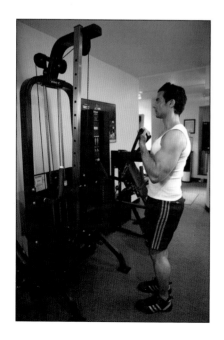

Using a weight that is 10 lbs. heavier than your 12 rep max, curl with one arm until you can't do another, then have your free hand help you into position so you can "lower" the remaining reps to make up 12.

Isn't that bicep exercise amazing! It doesn't even feel like you are doing any work, but wait until tomorrow when you can feel every fiber of your biceps. Many of my clients report more detail and better shape as soon as the next day after this workout.

High Intensity Tip

Add the High Intensity Cardio Kicker from Chapter Four to any of these workouts. By doing so, you'll still be finished and out the door in less than 30 minutes.

CHAPTER EIGHT: HIGH INTENSITY REST

Let's face it, some of the greatest things that happen to me happen in my bed or on my couch . . . sleep and naps. You may be thinking, *But this is a workout book… why is he talking about sleep?* To get the best results from these workouts, you will need time to recover. The importance of a good, restful, and sound sleep is underrated. It is an equal part of a two part equation: the workout (or stimulation) and the recovery process. If either one of these components is not up to snuff, the whole program is not going to come close to giving you all that it can.

Here's the deal. Poor quality or lack of sleep has been linked to:

Chronic Pain or Fibromyalgia

Weight Gain

Diabetes

Heart Disease

It has also been recently linked to Alzheimer's disease.

And this is just what we know about now. What other diseases do you think researchers will link poor sleep to? Don't take any chances; get a good night's sleep. If you have trouble sleeping, there are many options for you. Here are a few basic tips to try first.

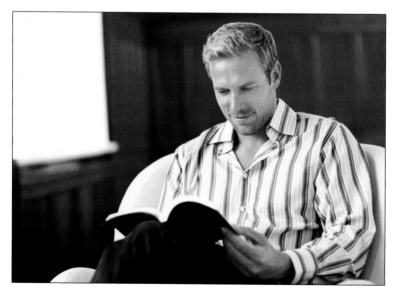

Time to kick back

Reduce caffeine intake	You may want to start by cutting back from two cups a day to one, or possibly cutting out that afternoon cup. It could be the caffeine that you have in the afternoon or evening that is throwing you off. If that doesn't help, try switching to decaf for a while and see if that does the trick.
Don't eat chocolate at night	Dark chocolate is a healthy snack, but there is some caffeine in it, so it's best not to have any right before bed. Anytime one of my clients tells me they didn't sleep well the night before, I always ask if they ate chocolate before bed. Ninety percent of the time, the answer is "yes."
Avoid an "energy boost" after 8:00 p.m.	Sugar and sugary foods will give you an energy boost. That can be useful right before a workout, but not right before bed. If you were thinking about a big bowl of cereal before turning in for the night—FORGET IT! So what to do?

Eat foods high in magnesium	Ever get knocked out by an almond? Almonds are high in magnesium and may be just the thing to take the edge off and knock you out for the night. Since it's a much better snacking alternative than what you may have tried tonight, give it a shot. Other foods high in magnesium are legumes, seeds (pumpkin seeds, sunflower seeds, etc.), dark leafy green vegetables, and cashews.
Take a pill	There are many options at the health food store. I suggest that you first try something, like L-Tryptophan or 5-HTP. These are basic, simple, and cost effective. You will best know what is working for you if you try single ingredient products as opposed to multi ingredient products.
Light reading	After you snack on some almonds and pop an L-Tryptophan capsule, how about a bedtime story to get you deep into a REM cycle. My favorite book about the benefits of sleep and the dangers of sleep deprivation is *Lights Out* by T.S. Wiley.

CHAPTER NINE:
HIGH INTENSITY NUTRITION

High Intensity Nutrition is just like the workouts—simple and straight to the point. One of the reasons that people fail at dieting is that they don't know where to start. Even worse, they'll try an overly complicated program and get so overwhelmed that they quit before they begin. Remember, this book is for the person who is tight on time and high on stress. If you have all day to grow your own organic vegetables after gathering fresh eggs from your hens, I would imagine I don't need to offer any advice to you. The rest of us, however, need a simple, no-nonsense plan. Enter Isagenix. If you have been following me on Facebook or Twitter all or read my first book (*The 90-Second Fitness Solution*), you know that I'm a believer in eating "real" foods, and always include whey protein in my diet. So why would I need Isagenix? It turns out that I really did need it and I should have known that. Let me tell you a story.

My Facebook friend Dee emailed and asked me to check out Isagenix, as she wanted my opinion about the products. I looked it over very quickly and emailed her back that it looked like one of those multi-level marketing companies and probably best to skip it. She told me that she was told the products were very good and that after trying them she felt great but would still feel better if I looked into it more closely. Normally, I would have dismissed Dee's claim that she "felt great" after using any product, but there is something that you need to know about Dee: She was a long-time vegan and the product she used was Isagenix Isalean Shakes, which were definitely NOT vegan. Now Dee had my attention! We set up a call and I couldn't believe that this company convinced her to go off the path of her vegan belief and try a whey protein product, especially since I preach the benefits of whey protein all the time to vegans and it always falls on deaf ears. Dee introduced me to Sherry Fox, and still being a skeptic, I signed up as an associate to see these products for myself. I knew that there was a chance that I'd be taken for a ride by another MLM scam, but I wanted to have a firsthand look at this stuff. Sherry, sensing my hesitation, set up a call with Tony Escobar so that I could ask him anything I wanted to know about the products and company. Tony called one night and the most amazing thing happened… I listened and learned! Look, I am a fitness professional for over 25 years. I've pretty much seen it all, heard it all, and tried it all. I very rarely run into someone that captures my attention and holds it the way Tony did that night. Within minutes I found myself grabbing a pad and pen and writing down words to look up, facts to research and notes that I didn't want to forget. It was amazing how knowledgeable he was of nutrition and exercise. The best part for me was that he is a former bodybuilder/ powerlifter like me, so we had a lot in common and went down many of the same diet and exercise paths. The bottom line is this: IsaLean and IsaPro protein come from "dairy cows that are raised on pastures (not grain fed) on small New Zealand family farms, milked according to season, well rested, and not treated with hormones or antibiotics." This is exactly what I want! I do not want my whey protein to come from grain-fed cows that are lined up by the thousands and abused while being pumped full of drugs! And it doesn't end there. I can get everything I need from Isagenix and don't need to go to a bunch of different stores and websites for the other things I need, like hemp seeds, fish oil, and supplements for joint support.*

---

* Contact me through my website petecerqua.com for more information.

I guess by now you figured out that I like Isagenix. No secret there. Here is how to use it for High Intensity Nutrition. The keys to a good nutrition program are simplicity and consistency. If you have no idea how many calories you are taking in or how much protein you're getting, how can you possibly know what changes you need to make? The first thing I do to get people on track is to get one meal at a time under control. These small changes will lead up to a big result and last much longer that going "all out" on a fad diet that will make you gain more weight than you lost after you bail on it.

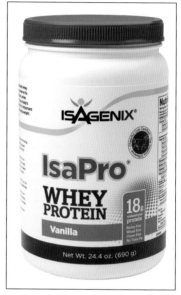

IsaPro Whey Protein from Isagenix.

Step One: Breakfast

While I'm sure you've heard it before, feeding your body properly first thing in the morning will set the tone (and your appetite) for the rest of the day. I have been promoting fresh vegetable juices with whey protein added or just a basic whey protein shake. My message stays the same, but this time I want you to try an IsaLean Shake or add IsaPro to your vegetable juice because of the reasons mentioned earlier. To make this plan work, you will have to commit to having a protein drink for breakfast at least six out of seven days per week. Feel free to change flavors or spice up the shakes a little as long as you don't change the caloric intake very much. It will benefit you to know that you are getting the exact same amount of calories each morning and that it only took a few minutes to get the job done. You will have the choice of shaking these up with a shaker or making your shake in a blender so that you can throw in a banana or some frozen berries. Either way, get into the routine!

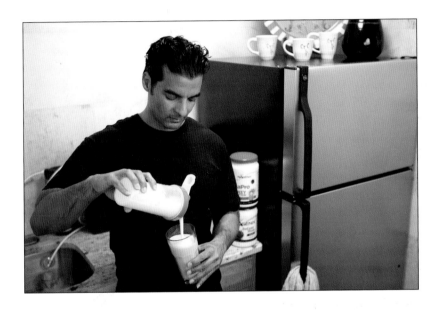

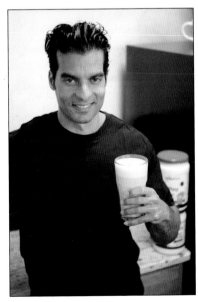

A shake for breakfast—easy.

Not in the mood for a Shake today?

Try an egg white omelet loaded with veggies a few days per week. You can be creative with the veggie combinations that you use each time or stick with a recipe that you like and look forward to. Whatever you do, do not go for oatmeal or cereal for breakfast, as it will only add to your "spare tire!"

Step Two: Lunch

If you are like me, you probably sit down to a relaxing three course meal for lunch at one of the finer restaurants in your area. Seriously, I'm moving like a freight train with no brakes all day. No time for a sit-down. It's going to have to be quick and painless. I have two options for lunch that fit me best and will serve you as well, a monster salad or a second protein drink. Half of the week I go across the street and get a chopped salad at the salad bar. You can't overdo fresh veggies so load up. Add a little protein like tuna, salmon, chicken or egg whites and you have a complete meal. Where people go wrong is the dressing. Some of the dressing options have more calories than a steak dinner. Don't fall prey to this big salad scam—get sensible. Opt for a basic oil and vinegar (not too much) or my favorite which is lemon juice. Again, the key is consistency so try to stick with the same program more often than not.

Option number two is a second protein drink. Usually I do 1 scoop of IsaLean with 1 scoop of IsaPro. Since you may not know the make-up of these two products, IsaLean is a good combination of protein and carbs, and IsaPro is all protein. I like to "lean" (pun intended) towards a little more protein, so one scoop of each will tilt the scales toward higher protein. You can do two scoops of IsaLean just as effectively, the choice is yours. Whichever route you choose, stick with it for at least a month so you can see how the program is working before making adjustments.

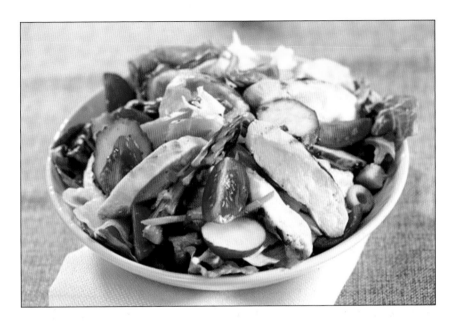

Another lunch option that I use each week is to have a Quinoa salad. Prepare the Quinoa over the weekend so you can simply scoop some into a bowl. Add chopped veggies along with some fresh parsley, cilantro, or basil. I usually add half of an avocado diced. Chopped walnuts or sunflower seeds optional. For a dressing:

2 Tbsp freshly squeezed lemon juice
2 Tbsp olive oil
¼ tsp salt
Fresh ground pepper

The Grand Finale: Dinner

Last meal of the day can be disastrous if you aren't careful. Scenario one is where you starved yourself all day and the only thing you consumed was Starbucks. This is bad. Your blood sugar levels are bouncing all around because you are living on high calorie caffeine with whipped cream all day, so the next meal you have will be converted to body fat since your body thinks it's starving. Scenario two is 80 percent of your dinner consisted of "the bread basket" and a nice chardonnay. I love the logic with scenario number two because people usually have dessert in this situation since they fell off their diet with the bread and wine. Keep it simple. Free range chicken or wild caught salmon with a vegetable and a salad is all you need. Remember that there are 21 meals in a week and you have to get 20 of them right to get rid of unwanted fat, so why not have a program laid out for you that lets you know exactly what to reach for when you are hungry? Well, I just did it for you. So try it, follow it, and embrace it! It will work, I promise.

High Intensity Tip

Whatever you choose for dinner, whether it be chicken, fish, or beef, make sure that the chicken and beef is grass fed and the fish is wild caught. This is very important to your health.

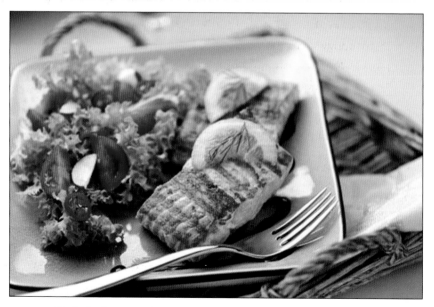

Grilled salmon steak with fresh salad and balsamic vinegar sauce.

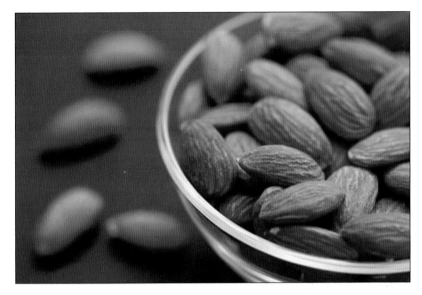

Raw almonds are a healthy snack that will keep you from reaching for the cookies.

The benefits of Grass Fed vs. Grain Fed:

Meat from grass-fed cattle is lower in artery-clogging saturated fat.
Grass-fed meat is higher in omega-3 fatty acids (Omega 3's are good
for us and we want them).
Grass-fed meat is four times higher in vitamin E.
Last but not least-grass-fed meat is higher in conjugated linoleic acid
(CLA), a nutrient associated with lower cancer risk and is also known
to reduce bodyfat!

Snacks

Snacking between meals does not have to sabotage your diet. In fact,
keeping your blood sugar levels balanced all day will help you stay on program. Some options would be a handful of nuts or a small piece of dark
chocolate. Make sure that you eat something every three hours, whether
it's a meal or a snack. I personally use one of many superfoods as my

snacks. Superfoods are high nutrient foods that will satisfy your appetite while improving your health. Feel free to mix and match until you find the Superfoods that will take the edge off. Remember portion control. Just because Superfoods are a healthy snack . . . it doesn't mean you can eat as much as you want. A handful or a cup will do in most cases.

A short list of Superfoods includes:

- Apples
- Avocado
- Blueberries
- Carrots
- Cherries
- Dark Chocolate
- Nuts (raw unsalted almonds and walnuts)
- Seeds (especially pumpkin and sunflower)
- Greek Yogurt

Hydration

I know, I know, you think I'm going to tell you to drink some ridiculous amount of water each day. I'm not. When did we become this super hydrating, water consuming society? Drink and pee, drink and pee, all day long. It's exhausting. If you're overheated and exercising too much, than I see the need for an increased amount of water. However, if you're following my program and getting your strength workouts in around 10 minutes, than you probably are not even sweating, so why would you need a gallon of water a day? I am 6'2" tall and weigh around 220 lbs. and I drink exactly one quart a day. No more, no less. If I feel dehydrated, I add a 16 ounce carton of coconut water to my schedule. Coconut water is high in potassium which is very good for the body. It is necessary for the heart, kidneys, and other organs to work normally. We usually do not get adequate amounts of potassium in our diet, so getting it from coconut water is a great idea, as it will hydrate and give added potassium. Popular brands of coconut water are Vita Coco, Zico, and Naked Coconut Water. I feel that there is the possibility of drinking too much water and that if you do, you will flush valuable nutrients out from your body. As you can see from my program and philosophy in general, I believe that "too much or too little" are no good. The goal is to get what you need. No more, no less.

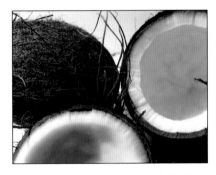

Coconut water is a great way to hydrate.

It is with great pleasure that I give to you *The High Intensity Fitness Revolution*. I hope the information provided will open your eyes to a new way of thinking about your health and fitness program.

Yours in Strength and Health,

Pete Cerqua

ACKNOWLEDGEMENTS

This book would not be possible if it were not for the love, support, and friendship of some very special people in my life:

Marylou Cerqua and Pete Cerqua, Sr.

A.k.a. Mom and Dad. Thank you for laying the groundwork and foundation of morals and principles that helped me build a business and raise a son. I love you both very much.

Gregg Stebben

Thank you for your friendship. You are the person that got the ball rolling on this book and opened doors for me. Whether you are on the East Coast or West Coast, it's nice to know you are close by.

Tony Lyons

I am honored to be a Skyhorse author. Thank you for the opportunity to be a part of the fastest growing independent publishing house in America and welcoming me to the Skyhorse family.

Jason Katzman

Thank you for your guidance and wisdom, without which this book would not be possible.

Tony Escobar

Your motivational skills are matched only by your wealth of knowledge. Thank you so much for sharing your knowledge and friendship. Every team needs a leader, but you are so much more. Thank you for motivating me and for welcoming me to your Isagenix family with open arms.

Sean Escobar

It's a great feeling to know that you are always a phone call or email away. Thank you for being there and for paving the way for me. Watching you lead by example both personally and professionally is truly an inspiration.

Dee Greenberg

Thanks Dee for your support and enthusiasm for my 90-Second Fitness program, and for introducing me to Isagenix. You inspired me with your story and experience and opened my eyes to the next level.

Sherry Fox

Your kindness and patience was very thoughtful and did not go unnoticed. Thank you for answering my questions and for your kind words and enthusiasm for my workouts.

Stefan Pinto

Thanks for traveling 3,000 miles when I needed you. I had you in mind for this project right from the start and hoped that it would work out. You are a great friend and I am so proud of your accomplishments.

Dara Jewett

Thank you for taking my vision and making it visible for all to see. Your flexibility, professionalism, and artistic design are unmatched.

The Gym Source

Friends for over 20 years! Thanks to Rich Miller and Nigel Anderson for letting us shoot at your NYC flagship location. When I met you both in 1988, you had a desk for each of you, a small showroom, and one location. Twenty-four years and 30 locations later, you are the gold standard for home and gym exercise equipment. I am proud to know you both.

90-Second Fitness Trainers

I am very fortunate to be working with close friends on a daily basis: Rob Federico, Anton Thompson, Jolynn Baca Jaekel, Alvin Rodriguez, Evelyn Hatzigeorgiou, James Lee, and Rick Swanson. All masters at their craft and great sounding boards. Thank you.

Pete's Army

Thanks guys for letting me push you through some great workouts: Alex Bici, Nick Giordano, Bob Friedman, Jason Giessel, PFC Matt Haiken, Alan Hartman, Bob Holland, Perry Jacobson, Chris Kern, Doug Smith, Tony Kolev, Steven Koppel, Bob Lerner, Larry "Dr. Muscles" Liebman, Robert Lipner, Bob Mann, Louis Rousso, Jay Schoenfeld, Jerry Shallo, Robert Simpson, Joe Spiegel, Oliver Stanton, George Whiteley, Ron Wilford, Glenn Chernoff, and Marty Wolff

Also Available in Vook Format from Vook.com

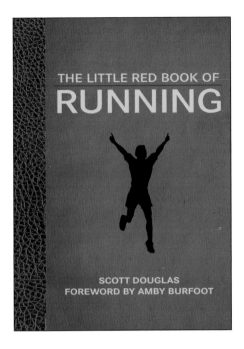

The Little Red Book of Running

by Scott Douglas

Foreword by Amby Burfoot

Scott Douglas offers the advice he's gleaned from three decades of running, from twenty years as a running writer, and from the deep connections he's made with top runners and coaches around the country and around the world. The 250 tips offered here are the next best thing to having a personal coach or an experienced running partner. Douglas includes tips for increasing your daily, weekly, and yearly mileage; advice on increasing your speed and racing faster; useful knowledge on how to stay injury-free and be a healthy runner; and much more.

The range of tips means there's something for any runner—someone looking to start running to get in shape, a competitive high school or college runner, an athlete looking to move into running, or an experienced runner looking to improve his or her time in an upcoming marathon. You have the questions: What running apparel is best? What kind of gear do you need to run in the rain or snow? How do you find time in a busy schedule to run? How can you set and achieve meaningful goals? Douglas has the answers.

$16.95 Hardcover

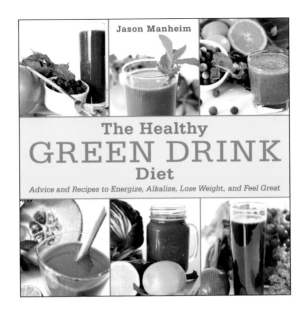

The Healthy Green Drink Diet

Advice and Recipes to Energize, Alkalize, Lose Weight, and Feel Great

by Jason Manheim

One juice or smoothie a day—made from green vegetables such as kale, cucumber, celery, and spinach—works wonders for organ health, immune system strength, and weight loss. Now the founder of heathygreendrink.com offers a persuasive argument for adding a green drink to your day, as well as recipes for dozens of different variations. Why drink green?

- Green leafy vegetables are extremely alkaline and great for lowering your blood pH and remedying many common ailments and diseases.
- By juicing or blending the vegetables into a delicious smoothie, you can enjoy the goodness of many more cups of greens that you could possibly eat in one sitting.
- The juicing process also breaks down or removes the fibers of the plants so their nutrients are able to get into your system quicker.
- The "green drink" approach offers dieters the chance to add something rather than take it away, without guilt.

The Healthy Green Drink Diet gives health enthusiasts all the tools they need to add green drinks to their daily routine and feel the wonderful, energizing results through and through.

$16.95 Hardcover

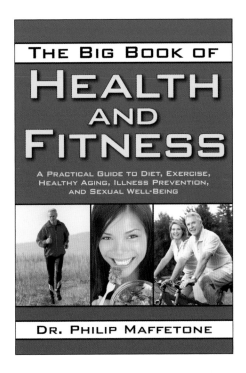

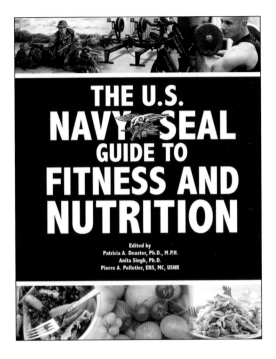

The U.S. Navy SEAL Guide to Fitness and Nutrition

Edited by Patricia A. Deuster, Anita Singh , and Pierre A. Pelletier

Developed for Navy SEAL trainees to help them meet the rigorous demands of the Naval Special Warfare (NSW) community, this comprehensive guide covers all the basics of physical well being as well as advice for the specific challenges encountered in extreme conditions and mission-related activities. Topics covered include calculating energy expenditure; definitions, functions, and daily allowances of carbohydrates, fats, and protein; nutritional considerations for endurance and strength training activities; active recovery from injury; cardio-respiratory conditioning; appropriate gear for running and swimming for fitness; exercising in extreme and adverse weather; and more. Compiled by physicians and physiologists chosen for their knowledge of the NSW and SEAL community, this manual is a unique resource for anyone wanting to improve his or her health, strength, and endurance.

$16.95 Paperback